Risk Matters in Healthcare
Communicating, explaining and managing risk

Foreword

Sir Kenneth Calman

Vice-Chancellor
Durham University
Former Chief Medical Officer

Radcliffe Medical Press

Radcliffe Medical Press Ltd
18 Marcham Road, Abingdon, Oxon OX14 1AA

British Library Cataloguing in Publication Data

A catalogue record for this book is available from the British Library.

ISBN 1 85775 456 5

Typeset by Advance Typesetting Ltd, Oxfordshire
Printed and bound by TJ International Ltd, Padstow, Cornwall

Contents

Foreword

Risk is a topic that is currently being discussed by a wide range of groups – professional, public and political. Doctors are no exception and general practice has its own range of issues in relation to risk. This book is described by the authors as a book in two halves, and to stretch the football analogy further there is an excellent review of definitions, strategy and tactics followed by a practical session on the field of play. A particularly interesting section is the one on comments by doctors on their thoughts on communicating risk. These feedback responses are both illuminating and full of educational messages. They set the context for much of the rest of the book.

For many years attempts have been made to create a 'risk scale', which would be of value to patients, the public and professionals alike. This book reviews a number of such scales and outlines their positive and negative features. The authors propose a 'risk ready reckoner', which chooses a series of clinical problems from breast cancer, amniocentesis and oral contraceptives to other medical interventions, and links them to risk estimates, a verbal description of the risk and a comparative. This is a most useful chart and will provide a helpful source of advice for doctors and other health professionals.

The second part of the book is about changing the culture and improving the management of clinical risk. There is an interesting discussion on common areas of risk in general practice. Two particularly good examples of personal and practice development plans in the area of clinical risk are stimulating to read and to learn from.

In conclusion, reverting to the football analogy, this book not only sets out some rules and provides general coaching, but is linked with 'on-the-pitch' experiences. It shows how to avoid penalties and how to score goals, all for the benefit of patients and the community. I enjoyed reading it very much.

Kenneth C Calman
October 2000

Preface

Like a football match, this book is in two halves. In Part One, we concentrate on defining risk and the factors influencing individuals as they make decisions about risk. Part Two deals with clinical teams making decisions about organisational matters and the working environment.

To effectively guide patients as they make decisions involving risk, we need to be aware of the risks posed by clinical and organisational situations, and also how best to communicate that to patients and colleagues for effective risk management. Health professionals 'have a responsibility to make a much greater effort to ... help the public by putting the levels of risk into context and ... enable people to judge ... significant levels of risk'.[1] This book demonstrates how those in the NHS can improve how they help patients share in decision making about their treatments from an informed standpoint.

Some patients want better information so that they can take more responsibility for their own care and make informed judgements about relative risks. Some doctors and nurses are trying to inform patients so that they can understand more about their illnesses, share in decision making about treatment and management options, and take more responsibility for their own health and wellbeing. Current resources for patient information/education/communication and understanding of risks is of variable quality or non-existent. People are calling for input into local and national decision making in the NHS. The book considers how this can happen in a meaningful way.

The emphasis is on practical aspects of how to explain risks to patients, what health professionals can actually do themselves to provide good-quality information and to understand the extent to which individual patients and the public need to be involved before they can make meaningful and informed decisions. We have tried to summarise some of the everyday information on risks that might be needed for discussions with patients and suggest ways in which that information might be conveyed, in response to our conversations with colleagues.

Risk management is an essential component of clinical governance. Risk assessment, risk reduction and risk management are all covered with respect to the practice organisation and working environment.

Kay Mohanna
Ruth Chambers
October 2000

---

1   Lomer G (1998) Risk assessment. *The Times*. 15 Sept (letter).

About the authors

Kay Mohanna has been a general practitioner for seven years, and is a lecturer in medical education at Staffordshire University. Kay teaches undergraduate epidemiology and medical ethics to medical and dental students. Her initial interest in how people evaluate risk and then use that information to make decisions was sparked during research considering a proposal for a compulsory community mental health treatment order. This was the basis of her Masters degree in medical ethics. Since then she has looked at how an understanding of risk affects the consent process as it involves pregnant women being asked to participate in clinical trials.

She has watched with interest the way the general public has been informed by the lay press about everyday risks involving diet, medicines and lifestyle. As a doctor, she is used to trying to translate scientific risk into meaningful discussions with patients and helping them to personalise that risk for themselves and their situations. She is interested in the question 'So what would that mean if it happened to me?' as well as 'How likely is that to happen?'

Ruth Chambers has been a general practitioner for 20 years and is currently the Professor of Primary Care Development at the School of Health, Staffordshire University. She became interested in involving patients and the public in decision making about the planning and delivery of NHS services while Chair of the Staffordshire Medical Audit Advisory Group and, later, author of her district's primary healthcare strategy. Personal experience of caring for a terminally ill child has given her an insight into how distressing it is for parents to be excluded by doctors, nurses and others in authority from involvement in important management decisions that involve risks in an individual's management.

Ruth has initiated and run all types of educational initiatives and activities. She has run workshops to teach GPs, hospital consultants, nurses, therapists and non-clinical staff about clinical governance. The experiences of the workshops and how the participants put their learning about clinical governance into action inform the second part of this book.

Acknowledgements

Much of our initial thinking about communicating risks originated from the published works of, and later conversations with, Professor Sir Kenneth Calman, Dr Peter Bennett and Dr Geoffrey Royston. We were able to consolidate and test much of our thinking at the Royal College of General Practitioners' millennium Spring Meeting at Crieff, where one of the themes was 'risk'.

The basis of the integration of risk management into a clinical governance culture that is central to the second part of this book was developed in a previous publication and through associated workshops for doctors and other health professionals with Dr Gill Wakley.[1]

We should like to acknowledge the contribution of all these experts in the field and the health professionals who have told us how they manage and communicate risk in their everyday practice. We should also like to thank the several taxi drivers and other members of the public who knowingly entered into conversations about risk to inform this book.

Finally, we hope that the risks we took with our relationships with families and friends by closeting ourselves away writing this book are at least equal to the benefits to you, as readers, in helping to increase your understanding of risk and risk management.

1   Chambers R and Wakley G (2000) *Making Clinical Governance Work for You.* Radcliffe Medical Press, Oxford.

PART ONE

Understanding and talking about risk

CHAPTER ONE

Risk: what's that all about then?

When it comes to risk management – everyone is an expert.[1]

We all automatically, maybe even subconsciously, make decisions in our daily lives that take into account the anticipated effect of likely outcomes. Often we are confident that we can predict the result of our actions and what it will mean to us if it does happen. Depending on our personality and our perception of risks and benefits, we will each make decisions that suit us and fit with the way we look at the world.

However, as Ulrich Beck acknowledged, risks can be 'changed, magnified, dramatised or minimised within knowledge and to that extent they are particularly open to social definition and construction'.[2] This subjectivity accounts for why there is such a wide variation in what we each consider to be 'risky' behaviour. Similarly, the results of previous 'gambles' – whether we survive or get our fingers burnt by our choices – will colour our judgement about the level of risk we perceive for a given situation.

So is it possible to produce one definition of risk that we would all recognise? We can say that:

risk is the probability that a hazard will give rise to harm.

Both the extent to which we judge that the harmful outcome is likely to occur and that to which we judge the likely outcome to be harmful, are subjective.

On the whole we tend to be overoptimistic about the risks we face. Most smokers acknowledge the connection between smoking and disease – although some, for a variety of reasons, deny it – but the extent to which they feel that risk applies to them is generally underestimated. Similarly, individuals tend to feel that advice about healthy eating and lifestyle applies to others. If asked to estimate the risk we feel that we face from heart disease, for example, or being involved in a car accident, there will be a bias towards optimism. Outcomes with a high probability tend to be underestimated. Interestingly, the risk we consider ourselves to be under from rare events, such as nuclear accidents, HIV, AIDS or bovine spongiform encephalopathy, tends to be overestimated.

So a misperception exists: a tendency towards the illusion of relative invulnerability, even complacency, where more common risks exist and one towards unnecessary concern for the less likely, but more newsworthy, events. Since perception of risk is a prerequisite for changes in behaviour, misplaced optimism may result in a barrier to preventative action. It is also true that the second type of error of perception can be a barrier to change. If we feel an increased sense of risk, especially when combined with low expectations for being able to deal with that risk, a 'helplessness reaction' may be provoked and obstruct intentions to adapt or modify behaviour. This has implications for the way doctors talk to patients about risk in an attempt to modify unhealthy behaviour.

In a similar way, some personality types will affect the way in which risk is allowed to influence our behaviour. Some people have a tendency to optimism despite the evidence. For pessimistic people, risks are assumed to be greater than they are, maybe as a self-protection mechanism.

All activity carries with it some level of risk; there is no such thing as absolute safety. Even so, our understanding and perception of the risk is influenced by our values and our experience. The value we place on our independence might colour how risky we feel it is to travel alone on the London Underground at night for instance, especially if 'everyone I know does it and has never come to any harm'.

Even though it is clear that our values colour our thinking about risk, this cannot fully explain how it is that certain outcomes are less acceptable to the extent that we will take action to avoid them, even if very unlikely, or not take other actions that would result in clear benefits. An additional complication is that focusing on values is not in keeping with the usual situation where we are often asked to *choose* between alternatives rather than *propose* our ideal alternative for any course of action. Proponents of value-focused thinking, however, encourage us to consider *values*, not *alternatives*, in decision making as a starting place to understand difference.[3] Our patients may tell us that although we may have all the statistics about risks of medical interventions, we don't know how it applies to them in their circumstances. (In fact they may be wrong about doctors' understanding of the statistics as well! More about that in Chapter 2.)

Consider a proposal to reduce fatalities in car accidents. Setting a speed limit of 20 miles per hour would reduce the number of crashes relative to a speed of 60 miles per hour. Such proposals, being put forward for inner cities, meet with strong opposition because they involve conflicting values – only one of which is reducing the number of deaths. Others have to do with convenience, saving time, cost and lost opportunities to do other things with the time that would be spent on the road. Since we almost certainly do not all hold identical value systems, this can result in decision making that others find difficult to comprehend. Proposals to decrease the speed limit on seemingly safe roads may infuriate those who drive for a living, such as lorry drivers and sales representatives. So in healthcare, just as in any other field, anticipated costs as well as benefits are taken into account by patients and interpreted in the light of what that outcome would mean to them, as they consider their options.

The extent to which we will tolerate the suspicion of risk then, is influenced by our preconceptions and beliefs, and our awareness of possible outcomes. We are influenced by what we see and hear. If a plane falls out of the sky, it will be reported on the news. The millions of successful flights each year go unmarked. A skewed or distorted image of the safety of aeroplanes as a form of transport can develop. Many people happily play the lottery every day without any idea of the 'risk' of winning the jackpot, spurred on by the success of friends and relatives winning ten pounds. Many continue to smoke, ever mindful of Uncle Fred who smoked till he was 98 years old and was knocked over by a bus on his way to the pub.

Availability bias leads us to overestimate the likelihood of future events happening if we have had similar events drawn to our attention, perhaps by the media. *Confirmation bias* results when new evidence is made to fit our understanding of how common an event is or our actions result in a self-fulfilling prophecy. Consider how often we have bought a new car only to suddenly notice them everywhere or how the experience of a miscarriage causes women to see pregnant women around every corner.

The understanding of how the world works, which guides our judgements about risk, might be described as background abstractions – paradigms, ideologies or beliefs – the set of shared assumptions that are formed through shared experience and that go unchallenged by those with whom we come into contact. The 'fallacy of misplaced concreteness' (wrote the philosopher Alfred North Whitehead in 1932) is the misperception that arises from confusing reality with one's abstractions. The analogy of winning the lottery, sometimes used by doctors in an attempt to try and clarify or interpret the likelihood of certain outcomes for patients, can be subject to such a fallacy. A doctor who describes a rare outcome as 'one in a million, like winning the lottery' may be saying that there is a very small but measurable risk of a particular outcome. If that outcome is death, then some patients would want that information to weigh against the benefits. However, the doctor could be saying, or the patient may interpret what is said as, 'that risk is so small it will never happen and is not worth considering'. Since the understanding of most lottery players of their likelihood of becoming a millionaire overnight is already delusional, the comparison is subject to the same misinterpretation.

A cautious person is likely to respond with diminished perception of the rewards of risk taking and a heightened perception of the adverse consequences of risk. This perceptual shift is mimicked in reverse for those considered by the cautious person to be reckless. Each would consider the other to be misjudging the outcomes, both good and bad, of an activity. This is brought into focus when we consider the opposing positions a seven-year-old and his mother would take about ice skating on a frozen pond.

Cultural theory

In an attempt to shed some light on the connection between 'culture' and an understanding of risk and subsequent risk-taking behaviour, cultural theorists consider one of the more popular models describing personality types. Here culture is described as the total map of our experience: the way we look at the world, what we have learnt from events in our lives and what we use to make sense of what happens to us.

Like all such models that attempt to categorise us into types, it is subject to the usual limitations. We may feel from the descriptions that we fall into different 'boxes' at different

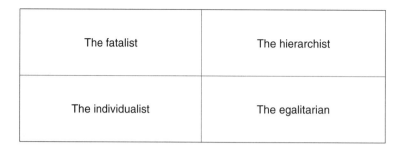

The fatalist	The hierarchist
The individualist	The egalitarian

Figure 1.1:   The cultural theory model of personality.[3]

times of the day or month, or depending on the circumstances or decision to be taken. The usefulness of a model like this depends on how accurately it can predict how we will act in a given set of circumstances. Cultural theorists, however, have tested out this model in different settings to demonstrate how robust it can be.

Moving along the horizontal axis from left to right in Figure 1.1, human nature becomes less individualised and more collectivist. People on the left of the spectrum may be less good at being members of a team but could be either leaders or eccentric geniuses. Moving towards the right, individuals become more interactive, they may structure the world into those at the top and those at the bottom of the pecking order; good 'foot soldiers' for example, as they recognise the individual contribution to the whole. Along the vertical axis, we move from behaviour described as prescribed – constrained by imposed restrictions and resulting ultimately in inequalities – to that which is not governed by any predetermined rules and where choices are governed by individuals resulting in more equality. In ideological terms, a parallel shift might be from communism to commune. Each has, in certain circumstances, both strengths and weaknesses. If we attempt to classify ourselves into these types, the position we occupy will represent powerful filters through which to consider the risks of life.

> Individualists are self-made people, free from control by others. They emphasise the individual responsibility to minimise personal risk, although they acknowledge the need for the development of social structures to allow collection and dissemination of information to facilitate this.

Individualists may perceive the risk of life as relatively stable, 'life is what you make it'. To be able to function independently, however, an individualist will recognise the responsibility of others to provide good information. They want the facts and then to be left alone to decide for themselves. These people are likely to ask themselves and their doctors, 'What has been the outcome of this intervention previously in people just like me?' They will have a strong sense of personal autonomy and resent any suggestion that the doctor knows best. In the role of doctor, the individualist may be more comfortable as an impartial giver of information – fine for individualist patients but less helpful for those requiring more guidance.

> Hierarchists inhabit a world of strong principle, with members knowing their place.

The hierarchist personality type is the total opposite of the individualist. For them what matters is the community experience and they will be more comfortable with public health issues, such as discussion of immunisation programmes. Honest reporting and knowledge gained by trial and error and experience may be seen as the best way to deal with risk at a community rather than a personal level. They need to minimise uncertainty in a discussion of risk with 'broad-brush' pictures and an epidemiological base to evidence. As a patient, they are likely to ask 'What is the general pattern among most people in my situation?' As the doctor, the hierarchist may feel that risk need not (or cannot) be individualised and therefore he or she will have difficulties with questions that require a tailoring of the known statistical evidence to the person in front of them, such as with questions like 'How do I know if that the 1 in 10 000 will not be me?'

> Egalitarians have a tendency to distrust 'experts' and the context within which risks are viewed is a social construct.

People who tend towards the bottom right in this model are the egalitarians, they have group loyalties and are led by the rules evolved within the group. Understanding and therefore avoiding risk can be improved by public participation as they try to work out from experience 'on the ground' what risks exist. They will be the patients who form patient participation groups and support groups. A doctor who tries to guide such patients towards his preferred treatment option will have less success than one who encourages the patient to search out others with similar conditions and compare notes about their experiences. A truly egalitarian doctor, however, may be good at jointly negotiating an understanding of risk with the individualist patient but less supportive of patients who need more guidance that they perceived as 'expert'.

> Fatalists diminish the importance of the group experience as a provider of evidence about outcomes and tend not to recognise the role of society as a force for change or a source of support.

A patient with a fatalistic approach may see life as a lottery, they may be resigned to their fate and see no point in trying to change it. The risks of life may be seen as part of the increasing complexity of modern life against which we have no defence. In consultation with doctors, they may decline preventative medicine or health promotion as part of their understanding that 'when your number's up, its up'. They are unlikely to perceive the benefits of hormone replacement therapy for example, considering the menopause a natural event that needs no intervention. This is not to say that they are likely to decline medical intervention, but that adverse outcomes are perceived as part of the swings and roundabouts of life. A claim for damages following a failure of sterilisation is unlikely to come from a fatalist. Doctors tend not to fall into this category, being trained in the 'cause-and-effect' model of medicine in which a diagnosis leads to a cure. But one who takes this approach may be less keen, for example, to refer patients for cosmetic surgery and may consider that risks such as bleeding, infection, scarring and anaesthetic hazards need stressing.

Even taking into account this variation in perception, it does not follow that the action of us all is to minimise the likelihood of harm resulting. Adams describes a 'risk thermostat'.[1] If by some means all risk could be removed from life, the theory states that we would be compelled to seek some activity that replaced the thrill of danger. To a greater or lesser extent we all build an element of uncertainty into our life to prevent boredom or to increase reward (Box 1.1). Our risk thermostat is not set at zero. As we take 'risks', we incur losses if harm results and rewards if harm does not result. Accidents are a consequence of risk taking and individual decisions are made as a result of a balancing act between the effects those accidents have on us and the value we place on the rewards.

Box 1.1:   The theory of risk compensation[1]

- everyone has a propensity to take risk
- this propensity varies from one individual to another
- this propensity is influenced by the potential rewards of risk taking
- perceptions of risk are influenced by the experience of accidental losses – one's own and those of others
- individual risk-taking decisions represent a balancing act in which the perceptions of risk are weighed against propensity to take risk
- accident losses are, by definition, a consequence of taking risk; the more risks an individual takes the greater, on average, will be both the rewards and the losses he or she incurs.

The setting of the thermostat varies from one individual to another and also for one individual over time. General safety measures introduced or the efforts made to reduce risk will not work if the measure does not affect people's propensity to take risks in the first place. If people drive faster when wearing seat-belts because they feel it is now safe to do so, the effect of the seat-belt law will not be to reduce overall risk. The thermostat is just readjusted upwards so that behaviour is modified, until we are back at a level of risk with which people were previously comfortable.

An additional factor that influences how we rate the acceptability of a risk, is the effect that that harm would have on us if it were to occur. Variously known as the 'dread factor' or 'fright factor', but which could also be described conversely as the 'jackpot effect', these can be more important than the statistical probability of occurrence. The risk of inducing a miscarriage after amniocentesis, at about 0.5–1%, is about the same numerically as the risk of trisomy 21 at a maternal age of 40 years and is two to three times greater than the risk of trisomy 21 for a 35-year-old woman (1 in 365). For some people, the possibility of a miscarriage would be an acceptable risk, whereas the risk of giving birth to a baby with Down's syndrome would not. This also helps to explain why people play the massive odds against winning the lottery: 'Wouldn't it be lovely if I did?'

Communicating risk

Since we can now see that people perceive risk differently and also that risk means different things to different people, we can see that there must be implications for the way in which we communicate risks to our patients. People will vary in their acceptance of risk however the balance of risk and reward is described. One individual may even vary over time, as circumstances and life events change. For example, as we become parents, we may not tolerate risks for our children, or for ourselves on behalf of our children, that we were prepared to accept for ourselves before we became parents. Patients may modify their own behaviour as this perception changes, rather than in response to the exhortations of the medical profession. On a public health level, legislation in particular is doomed to failure if the perception of the consumer does not match that of the people changing the rules. An example of this was the clear flouting of the rules governing the sale of beef on the bone in the UK in 1998. Butchers made such products available 'under the counter' and high-profile restauranteurs continued to supply the demand.

A second obstacle awaits the unwary Public Health Minister or Director of Public Health. The public needs to *trust* the source of information in addition to believing the magnitude of a risk. Government departments and official bodies, at times including the medical profession and 'scientists', are increasingly held in less esteem than might previously have been the case. Part of this is people's observation that doomsday predictions have failed to come true ('I had whooping cough as a child, it didn't do me any harm, why do I need to give my child a risky injection?'), but part of it is the failure to match information to what people need to hear, both in language and content.

It is important to avoid inducing a feeling of helplessness in a discussion of risk. A person who feels that change will have no effect on the inevitability of a poor outcome may be as unlikely to change as one who is unrealistically optimistic about his or her chances.

In view of these differences, it may be impossible to know what sorts and sizes of risk matter to patients, varying as it will from person to person and for one person over time. Attempts have been made, however, to establish some broad categories of anxiety-provoking outcomes (Box 1.2).[4] To some people at some time, items on this list will be more significant than others in the reaction that they are likely to provoke and the list may predict how groups of people will react in general. They are less useful however in predicting how an individual will react.

Box 1.2:   Fright factors[4]

Risks are generally more worrying and less acceptable if perceived:

- to be involuntary (e.g. exposure to pollution) rather than voluntary (e.g. dangerous sports or smoking)
- as inequitably distributed (some benefit while others suffer the consequences)
- as inescapable by taking personal precautions
- to arise from an unfamiliar or novel source
- to result from manmade rather than natural sources
- to cause hidden and irreversible damage, e.g. through onset of illness many years after exposure
- to pose some particular danger to small children or pregnant women, or more generally to future generations
- to threaten a form of death (or illness/injury) arousing particular dread, e.g. cancer
- to damage identifiable rather than anonymous victims
- to be poorly understood by science
- as subject to contradictory statements from responsible sources (or even worse from the same source).

Therefore we have already identified certain important factors that will influence the reaction of any individual to information on risk.

- The impact of the anticipated outcome must matter to the patient.
- Action required to influence such an outcome must fit his or her 'map of the world'.
- There must be agreement that such an outcome is possible. The source of the information must be trustworthy.

Measuring risk

When we try to quantify a level or risk we take from the language of gambling; in explaining the actual likelihood of potential outcomes we talk of *odds*. In the language of risk, this is *probability*, a statistical, mathematical concept. As a tool for helping people understand the implications of decisions they make, probability has its strengths and limitations. Because it follows the usual mathematical rules about combining probabilities, it can make predictions about two uncertain events difficult to envisage, such as, for example, future recurrence of cancer and the effectiveness of treatment if it does recur. The chance of someone who tests positive in a screening test for a rare disorder actually having that disorder is a function of the sensitivity and specificity of the test, a mathematical concept that can be complex to share with patients. The difficulties increase when we try to explain that screening for rare conditions in a low-risk population will lead to an increase in false positives.

It is not just patients who find understanding the measurement of risk complex. Probability has an in-built difficulty for anyone whose first language is not numbers. We can understand that a hundred-to-one outsider is less likely to win a horse race than the three-to-one favourite, but is a side effect of a drug with a risk of 1:10 000 something we need to be concerned about? What if there is a risk of death of 50% from that side effect. Or a 12% risk of impotence?

Changes in level of risk are also fraught with difficulty. The oral contraceptive scare in 1995 was provoked by talk of a 'doubled risk' of thrombosis for users of some third-generation contraceptive pills. The risk of thromboembolism in non-pill users is five cases per 100 000 women per year. The excess risk (compared with non-pill users) of venous thromboembolism in pill users is 5–10 cases per 100 000 women per annum. In the third-generation pills, this figure for excess risk increased to around 10–20 cases per 100 000 users. How can we interpret the level of risk that this represents to an individual woman? Talk of a 'doubled risk', however, led to women stopping the pill and reports of increases in the rates of terminations of pregnancy in some areas. Since the risk of thromboembolism in pregnancy is variously put at between six and 20 per 10 000 (and 1 in 100 postpartum), it is clear that the language of risk did not assist in rational decision making.

We need to understand the terms used to be able to extrapolate the meaning of a research paper and thus explain the risks and benefits to others. We need critical appraisal skills to be able to form an opinion as to whether we can depend on the results from a research study. For example, it is well known that subjects excluded from a randomised controlled trial tend to have a worse prognosis than those included, which limits the generalisability of the findings.

Risk management will involve understanding scientific terms about risk so that we do not misinterpret research findings and mislead others about their choices.

One potential area for confusion is the difference between *relative* and *absolute* risk. If we consider the benefits of an intervention such as treatment with drug X in two groups of patients, A and B, the differences between these two terms become clear. Consider the outcome of a treatment, perhaps reduction in fatal heart attacks in diabetics, in group A, which is given the treatment, and in group B, which is given an inactive placebo (or not diagnosed and not treated). The percentage reduction in heart attacks resulting from the treatment can be calculated by comparing the difference in the heart attack rate between groups A and B with what would have happened with no treatment, that is the number of heart attacks in group B. This reduction is in *relative* risk; the outcome in one group, relative to another. It is not tailored for any individual in that group.

There is, however, a risk attached to 'no treatment', which will vary from one individual to another. This will depend on how many other risk factors exist for that person, whether in group A, receiving treatment, or group B. For the person with coexisting risk factors, smokers or those with high blood pressure for example, the likelihood of a heart attack without treatment is greater. In terms of relative risk reduction, those with or without additional risk factors would benefit equally from drug X. The effect of treating a person with additional risk factors, however, may be to reduce his 'absolute' risk back to the level of the person without risk factors. The significance of such an absolute risk reduction for a person with additional risk factors is clinically more useful, since these patients are at a higher priority for treatment.

If we divide the same patients into group C, those with additional risk factors for heart attacks, and group D, those without, we can calculate the absolute risk of a poor outcome in the presence or absence of treatment for both groups. For group C, the incidence in the treated group subtracted from the incidence in those on no treatment, will be the absolute risk reduction and it will be greater than the same calculation for group D. The change in risk has now been tailored for the pre-existing state of the patient.

(One step further in this series of calculations is to divide the absolute risk reduction for each into one – take its reciprocal – and the result will be the number we need to treat in each group to prevent one heart attack. For those readers keen to pursue this further, see Sackett's description of the calculation of number needed to treat.[5])

For doctors studying the results of scientific investigations the talk of absolute or relative risk reduction can be complicated. For the patient it can be a minefield of potential confusion.

What would be worse, an action (such as a chemical spillage as waste is transported to a safe means of disposal) that caused an increase in deaths from poisoning by 10% or another risk exposure (such as emptying the waste into the local river in the usual way) that doubles the expected deaths from that cause? Clearly the answer is that it depends on how many deaths would otherwise be expected, the baseline probability of death from each action. Per 10 million people exposed, a 10% increase on a risk of 1 in 100 000 produces 100 extra deaths, whereas a doubling of a risk of 1 in 10 000 000 produces only one extra death.

Another clinical scenario where absolute and relative risk reduction are confused is the use of hormone replacement therapy. The relative risk of developing breast cancer after five years of hormone replacement therapy increases by 30%. Anything increasing by nearly a third sounds alarming, and patients and doctors alike may be wary of a risk described in those terms. The absolute risk, however, is very low and that 30% represents the difference between an absolute risk of 10% in the general population of women aged 50, with one of 13% for those taking hormone replacement therapy.[6]

Offering numerical advice may not reassure someone who has first-hand knowledge of a bad, though rare, outcome from a certain activity. In other circumstances, a description of the implications of an outcome may be more helpful to a patient who has less of a grasp of figures and regards rare outcomes as unimportant.

So do numbers matter? Increasingly, and rightly, consumer groups expect doctors to involve their patients in decision making, giving them all the information they need to make an informed choice. This is often interpreted as a requirement to share statistical information as well. But many doctors, let alone patients, can find numbers, probabilities and likelihood ratios difficult to interpret. How many of us would spot that the numerical example given above in relation to trisomy 21 means that at a maternal age of 35 years, amniocentesis could result in the loss of two or three normal fetuses for every diagnosis of Down's syndrome?

A familiar difficulty arises in genetics cases. The risk of a child inheriting a recessive condition if both parents are carriers is 25%, or one in four. It is not unheard of for parents to assume that after one affected child the next three would be healthy as they have 'used up all their bad luck'.

Framing effects

'There is nothing either good or bad but thinking makes it so.' So says Shakespeare through the medium of Hamlet. The way in which a consequence is presented is termed its frame and this can affect the choices we make, clouding or enhancing the true consequences of an action. The effect of an event depends on our starting point – whether our state after the event will be better or worse than it was at the beginning. The description of a good outcome can lead us to bet on the sure thing, to be *risk averse*, whereas if the outcome is presented as a loss, we tend to be *risk seeking* and gamble to avoid certainty.

This leads us to a careful consideration of the language we use to describe outcomes to patients. Would you choose an intervention with a 40% failure rate or a 60% success rate? The actual risk of the two interventions is the same, but many would choose the one 'framed' in terms of gains. Doctors use framing almost instinctively to discourage patients from certain activities, framing in terms of negative outcomes while still giving correct factual information.

Conclusion

Health professionals may feel that the public wants to move towards total abolition of risk and is becoming unable to tolerate either uncertainty of risk level or knowledge of medical risks. Perhaps patients have started to believe that we only have to work at it a bit harder and we will be able to make medicine risk-free.

Many doctors will recognise the anecdote of the patient who failed to take medication having read the drug company's safety leaflet inserted in the medication pack. A GP who defined such a response with a Read code and logged them as they occurred, measured a rate of non-compliance attributable to the 'scare' factor of the patient information leaflet equal to nearly half that of the 'did not attend' rate of missed appointments with

GPs in his practice.[7] Maybe this is an illustration of the increasing, unfiltered information about risk to which patients now have access. Being so inundated with information renders us unable to sort out which risks need action and which do not.

To make well-informed decisions it is important to have a clear understanding of what can affect our perceptions of the risks and benefits resulting from choices that we make. In addition, risk is most effectively managed by individuals if there is awareness of what the risks are and how they compare with each other. It is not logical to worry about the risks of life until you have compared the risks which concern you with those that don't, but perhaps should.

The man who decides to make a sponsored parachute jump for charity is choosing not to minimise risk but to take hold of it and use it to enhance other values of life, such as excitement and altruism. For that person, the decision to jump may have been made in ignorance of the risks or in spite of the risks. He may have perceived the risk just as we would and made a balanced decision based on his value system, or decided that the added danger enhanced the excitement. He might not value hobbies that do not offer a contrast to his dull job and consider those a waste of time. He may know someone who success-fully completed such a jump previously, thus skewing his perception of the safety of the activity, or have known someone injured in a similar activity and decided that it could never happen to him. He might modify his behaviour finding an explanation for the previous poor outcome that will not be repeated.

Our advice to patients must fit with the way they look at the world. An attempt to balance risks and rewards for patients is doomed to failure unless we take into account their personality and understanding. The language we use to describe risk is as important as the way we measure it and present it.

References

1   Adams J (1995) *Risk*. UCL Press, London.

2   Beck U (1992) *Risk Society*. Sage, London.

3   Keeney RL (1992) *Value Focused Thinking*. Harvard University Press, London.

4   Bennett P and Calman K (eds) (1999) *Risk Communication and Public Health*. Oxford University Press, New York.

5   Sackett D, Haynes RB, Guyatt GH and Tugwell P (1991) *Clinical Epidemiology: a basic science for clinical medicine*. Little, Brown and Co, Boston.

6   Edwards A, Elwyn G and Gwyn R (1999) General practice registrars responses to the use of different risk communication tools in simulated consultations: a focus group study. *BMJ*. **319**: 749–52.

7   Willis J (2000) *Risk in the Surgery: communicating risk to patients*. RCGP Spring Symposium, Crieff, Scotland, April 2000 (presentation).

CHAPTER TWO

Risk communication

Talking about risk with patients has always been an important issue for doctors, nurses and health visitors on a one-to-one basis. Whether we are talking about primary prevention, such as giving health promotion advice about lifestyle, or secondary prevention involving counselling about screening tests and immunisations or the risks and benefits of treatment options, we are involving patients in discussions about risk.

Psychological research has shown that though patients want to be informed, for example about potential complications of surgery, presenting this information is difficult. Difficulties of risk communication may be associated with the person conveying the information or the person receiving the information. Table 2.1 gives a summary of some of these difficulties.

Table 2.1: Difficulties associated with communicating risk to patients[1]

Doctor factors	Patient factors
Doctors present varying amounts of information depending on their assessment of the patient's educational level and the patient's age	About half of all information related to patients is forgotten
Doctors' own perception of risk varies	Levels of understanding have been estimated at between 7% and 47%
	Individuals find it hard to digest numerical representations of risk
	People have difficulty in assigning numeric values to probabilistic words

A study in a London teaching hospital in 1998–99 set out to investigate how accurately patients could recall information given to them in outpatients. Patients' perceptions of risk information was also assessed. A questionnaire was given to 30 patients awaiting coronary bypass grafting immediately after their consultation and was followed up three weeks later with another questionnaire conducted over the telephone.[2]

- Patients were better at estimating numerically their risk of death than the risk of morbidity.

continued overleaf

- Patients recalled approximately one-half to two-thirds of the information given to them.
- This information is retained over time.
- They recalled verbal information better than numeric information.

Given the increasing concerns over consent issues regarding patients who survive but suffer an adverse outcome, presentation of risk would appear to need supplementing to encourage patients to give more thought to the risks of morbidity. Representation of risk in probabilistic terms is probably not as useful as verbal or categorical (high/low) representation.

Increasingly, patients are becoming more enquiring, more exposed to information and are being encouraged to take an active part in the process of decision making for themselves. If we are to engage effectively with patients and ensure their fully informed consent for interventions or to effectively guide them about lifestyle choices, they will need good information delivered in a way that they can understand; we will need to give clearer and fuller descriptions of risk.

How many people do you know who have a personal computer at home and access to the World Wide Web? The quality of the information on the Internet is variable, but there is open access to all. It is estimated that 40% of the 10.6 million British Internet users have already logged on to health-related websites. Patients with chronic diseases often have support groups and may become better informed about their own medical conditions than some health professionals.

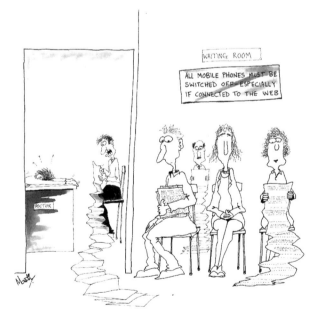

▼

'I don't think it breeds hypochondriacs. You always get those. There are often people sitting in postgraduate medical libraries who have no right to be there. How often do people come out of their doctor's surgery remembering the name of their condition but little else that the GP has said? A good medical website can enable them to go home, look it up and write down questions that they can ask the GP on the next visit.'

David Morgan, Honorary Senior Lecturer in Surgery, Birmingham, and co-founder of medicdirect.co.uk (*see* Appendix)

Websites for rare conditions often contain useful information, but they are unregulated and the information may at best be unavailable to all patients, unsuitable for some or even dangerous, particularly on treatment options. The fabled patient with a printout from the Internet is still quite rare, but when it happens we need to be able to guide them through the information and help them make informed choices.

If we did not already realise the need for this openness in discussion about healthcare issues, it was clearly illustrated in 1999, when a patient in America successfully brought a case claiming that she was not made aware of the chances and implications of a false negative result from a screening test.[3]

In a similar case, a British woman recently received an out-of-court settlement of £40 000 from a health authority, when she claimed that she had not been informed of possible outcomes of hormone replacement therapy. Her health problems, which may have included the breast cancer she subsequently developed, were not the basis of the claim but rather that she felt she had not been involved in the decision to have an implant at the time of her hysterectomy.

'It was not about the money it was about the principle of not being consulted. I didn't know anything about the effects it could have and I was told [when finding out about the implant] it would make me better. I believed what the doctors were saying.'

The 'mushrooming' of the amount of information available to patients has also brought a new opportunity to healthcare. We are in a better position than ever to build strong partnerships between health professionals and patients based on a shared understanding of clinical risks and benefits. Part of our responsibility towards our patients in the wider context should be to guide them to reliable sources of information. The British Medical Association (BMA) is putting together a website with validated data, and other sources are available (*see* Appendix).

The information technology subcommittee of the General Practitioners Committee of the BMA has drawn up a guide for patients wanting to use medical websites. Dr Paul Cundy, chairman, recommends:

- never rely on information from one site only
- check that quoted research has been published in a reputable journal
- check the site is updated regularly
- check for links to commercial organisations that might suggest bias
- avoid online consultations and diagnosis
- check whether the site respects confidentiality
- avoid sites claiming miracle cures
- seek out sites where the author is identified and credentials are listed
- look for sites with contact addresses, not email only.

There are difficulties lurking here for the unwary health professional. Patients are often anxious when we see them and may tend to rely on us to make decisions for them, especially if they are ill. The most independent person has been known to defer to his or her doctor with the words 'whatever you think best then doctor'. If we, as health professionals, accept this level of devolved responsibility for some, even those of us with the most patient-centred style are in danger of adopting a paternalistic attitude to other patients. This can lead us to the presumption that 'patients don't want to know all the ins and outs' and would like clear guidance on what we think they should do, as we shall see below.

Another challenge presented by the increased involvement of patients in decision making about their care, is the need for doctors to have a good grasp of the reality of the level of risk represented by certain actions or therapeutic interventions. Accurate data, clearly presented, are a prerequisite for effective patient involvement in decisions about their own health. Good data on risk are hard to come by in some cases. Knowledge of where to find and how to access the data is a skill we need to cultivate. This for some may be bound up with the idea of keeping up to date in general, but for others will involve specific searches for information to answer patients' questions.

Doctors talking

Risk scales are descriptive models to aid understanding of the probability of risk. Several have recently been proposed in the literature. The second part of this chapter describes and discusses some of these tools. However, none of these has yet been used in a controlled way with experienced doctors to see whether they enhance understanding, and many are not based on a consideration of what actually happens in consulting rooms at the moment.

Health professionals are experienced in describing and conveying an understanding of the likely outcomes of interventions in terms of harm and benefit, on an individual basis.

We thought it likely that health professionals have developed individual maps to assist them as they describe the territory of risk to their patients. To try to understand what is happening in consultations, we carried out a pilot study in Staffordshire. Informal conversations with colleagues helped us initially to clarify some of the issues for doctors.

Some GPs commented on the risk scales that they had seen to describe risk.

'The only useful one I can recall is the Margaret Pike figures about the risks of vascular complications of oral contraceptive pills, which uses a full Wembley Stadium as the denominator population. I always felt that wasn't so appropriate an example for women! The new cardiac risk scales are a good example of the complexity of such tools, difficult for professionals to understand let alone patients! Is 3% per annum the same as a 30% risk over 10 years? I think not, but I'm not certain how to explain!'

'The time I could do with something to describe risk is when I want to spell it out for a patient. I sometimes dig out a chart to make more impact. The cardiovascular risk scales (Framingham/New Zealand, etc.) make everyone's eyes glaze over, mine included, but I do use them to point out that wherever they are on the chart, stopping smoking makes a bigger difference than ANYTHING I can do!'

Fifteen GPs who had been in practice from between four and 30 years were engaged in in-depth discussions about risk and risk communication with patients. Their ideas and comments tended to group together into four main recurring themes throughout the interviews. We have termed these: patter, steering, interpreting and second opinion.

Doctors in this study relied on four main methods of dealing with the question of risk. Many doctors use more than one method in some consultations. The difficult subjects of relative and absolute risk, as well as helping patients make choices that are consistent with other aspects of their lives, have, over a period of time, led these doctors to develop individual ways of handling the consultation. All the following quotes in boxes are based on comments from real GPs talking about how they discuss risk with patients. Within each box, each quote is taken from a different doctor.

The patter

The first theme can loosely be described as the patter.

'It's the sort of thing you read in a paper at some stage and then it gets stuck in your head to be trotted out time and again. It becomes part of your patter.'

Most of the GPs interviewed have a favourite way to describe certain risks. They don't stop to think, they just launch into a familiar 'spiel'. If forced to reflect on what they are saying, they may realise that they no longer know the evidence base for their comments or even if the figures are correct. Indeed, they may never have known the facts about situations on which patients come to them for advice. They may not have seen the evidence first-hand but heard it in a lecture or in conversation with someone else. However, they continue to use examples or anecdotes that they find helpful or persuasive, either because those examples stuck in their mind or because they have found them helpful in conveying information to patients in the past.

'I use the one about the pill – the risk of dying is less than the risk of being killed crossing the road. I think it was in the John Guillebaud book and it sounded good and was easy to picture what it is about so I keep on using it.' [Guillebaud J (1993) *Contraception: your questions answered* (2e). Churchill Livingstone, London.]

'Recently I have been using numbers-needed-to-treat when talking about otitis media. I am already forgetting the numbers but it is something like we need to treat 17 children with antibiotics to make any appreciable improvements to symptoms for one child, but there is a risk of side effects (diarrhoea, rash and the like) of one in five. So little Johnny is usually better off without.'

'I saw something really useful on daytime TV. I say, "Do you know how dangerous smoking is? Tell me, of 100 smokers how many will die from it?" The answer is that 50 will die – so if there's two of you sitting here one will die. I have no idea how accurate that is or where the evidence came from for that, but it was startling and I remembered it.'

'I say about the pill and smoking. If you smoke then the potential risks of the pill are tenfold. I don't know if that's right exactly, it's just something that's easy to use and makes the point.'

'Take a classroom of 36 women. Three will get breast cancer; if they all take hormone replacement therapy you only need 33 women for three of them to get breast cancer. I think I got that from the local obs and gynae consultant.'

Steering

The second common theme can be described as steering. Some GPs in this study admitted to stressing risks in one direction or the other to influence the patient to take what they consider to be the 'right' decision.

'The main thing is that you are often trying to "sell" the treatment to the patient and you don't want to stress the bad side. You are supposed to give him information that will let him make an informed choice, what is likely to happen, but not the rare things or it will just put him off. You don't want to alarm them.'

'GPs are salespeople who sell health, so they skew the statistics and don't worry about the inaccuracy of the information they are giving to patients on risk if it sells health.'

For them the means – incomplete (or inaccurate) discussion of the risks – justified the ends: the patient agrees to take the treatment the doctor recommends or modifies his or her behaviour.

Often the language used was intentionally loaded to imply greater risk:

> 'When I'm talking to a teenager who is a smoker I explain the risks of smoking by saying: "Take you and three mates, if you all smoke 20 a day until you are 60 you might as well draw a straw for which of you will die from it." If you want people to change, it doesn't matter if it's a bit scary. Even the Department of Health puts up posters saying "Smoking Kills". It's not to frighten them – that's just a fact.'
>
> 'If she won't comply with treatment I might say that she has a risk of dying.'
>
> 'I read something about how to describe the risk of lung cancer to a teenager – it's no use saying you may get lung cancer in 40 years, because 40 years is hard to imagine. Instead you say you may have children one day and you don't want to leave them as orphans do you?'

Some would stress the risks of an option for which they themselves had less of a preference. One doctor described how he would present a discussion of risks heavily weighted towards a decision that suited the doctor better. At times in this conversation it became clear that that could even be so far as to be against a patient's best interests.

> 'Hormone replacement therapy creates a lot of extra work, what with the extra follow-up, more blood pressures to take and more referrals from the practice nurse. I tell them the statistics, e.g. I might say that three in 10 000 women might be saved from having a myocardial infarction, whereas three in 10 000 women might get breast cancer who wouldn't have had it. I think the risks are neutral, they balance each other out and the only reason women want to take it is to look younger for longer, whatever they say is the reason they want it.'

Interpreter of risk

A third, related theme was of the GP as interpreter of risk. Assumptions were made about what patients wanted and needed in a consultation. Some of the doctors interviewed said that patients 'are no good with numbers'. They felt that patients want, so they use, language such as 'high risk', 'low risk', 'increased risk'. Some said that patients did not want actual numbers, just a comparison or an idea of what the doctor thought their chances were.

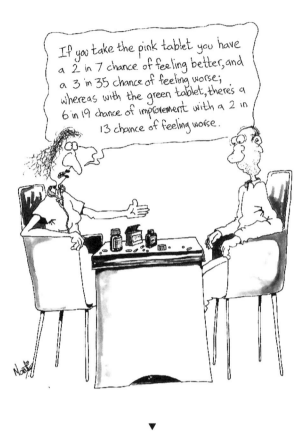

'Very few people need to know numbers. If I refer someone to be sterilised I might say that there is a theoretical risk of complications and describe what might happen. They may ask how common and I say one in 400. After that they never go any further. I don't think they know what one in 400 means though.'

'I try to make it black and white at the expense of oversimplification and loss of complete scientific validity. As a GP I am always interpreting risk for patients.'

'If he says, "what is my risk of getting prostate cancer before I'm 50", I say, "It's minimal, it's very rare." If he asks me to be precise I would say that I can't put a figure on it but I can say "Don't worry about it, it's a disease of old age".'

'They want to hear if you think it's likely, so I say things like, "You are a lot more at risk than the norm".'

'I have already read the evidence, done the thinking and can give them a potted version of it. Patients don't want details and sometimes it's hard to get them involved in the discussion. They are quite willing to do what the doctor thinks is best.'

Some doctors considered that it was not only patients who had problems understanding and remembering numbers:

> 'People don't think in terms of odds ratios, they want problems sorted. I wouldn't try to explain the risks and benefits of antibiotics in otitis media because I can't remember all the pros and cons. I would just give the prescription. Acting on that basis makes a compassionate doctor, but I suppose it is not evidence-based. The balance between risk and benefit is hard though. When people are in pain you want to try anything just on the off chance that might help.'

The same doctor said:

> 'OK, let's take hormone replacement therapy and breast cancer. If a woman pins me down to a number I might say "Well if you take HRT you, what is it, double your risk is it? In round figures anyway. If you have not got a close family history of breast cancer you will have to weigh that risk up for yourself".'

Second opinion

Finally, those in this study described a fallback option. If all else fails you can get a second opinion.

If patients are keen for hard facts these doctors dealt with this by searching for the evidence themselves or referring to a hospital consultant. If the discussion about therapy options got too hard there was always the option to admit for initiation of treatment.

> 'If a man needs surgery and wants to know what his risk of impotence or incontinence is I will chicken out and tell him to ask the specialist at the clinic. I would say that it is a problem, but it's not inevitable, but I can't quantify it. You couldn't say there's definitely not a risk because that would be deceptive. So you need a word between possibly and likely and words mean different things to different people. I would opt for 'low risk'. You don't want to frighten people off the op. But the specialist will have the numbers at his fingertips because his specialty is more narrow.'
>
> 'Once, when the balance of surgery was very fine, I rang the consultant and we discussed it then I got the patient back and we went over it. As a GP you are acting as the go-between more often than you think.'
>
> 'I tried and failed to explain to a Polish lady the risks and benefits of taking an ACE (angiotensin-converting enzyme) inhibitor for her failure. In the end I just admitted her through casualty.'
>
> *continued overleaf*

'I sent one woman to the obstetrics department to ask some questions we had worked out. I didn't know the chances of a vaginal delivery for a breech. The obs registrar said "I could tell you but you wouldn't understand". I told her that she should have said "Don't you think it's your job to explain it to me so that I can understand?"'

Our own favourite in this section was:

'If anyone ever asked me for the number-needed-to-treat that would be a real indication to refer them to the outpatients.'

The GPs in this pilot study took their role as information giver very seriously and many had thought about how to talk about risk already. There was a feeling though that patients do not need actual figures but rather that the GP should be able to understand and interpret their risk. Many of the doctors happily stated that a knowledge of true facts about absolute risk was not necessary either for the doctor or the patient. Some pointed out that the concept we need to get across to patients was that they had a choice, being seemingly oblivious to the fact that without the facts, patients would be in a poor position to make such a choice.

Two contradictory reasons were given for why GPs did not need to know the absolute facts about risk. First, there was a tendency to steer away from the general facts in the belief that when patients come into their consulting room they expect a personal consultation about their health. They want to know: What is the actual risk to me? How do I know if I am that one in 10 000 that you are talking about?

Other GPs felt that data were not needed because patients couldn't understand them anyway. It was interesting that doctors in this survey said that at times they would try to steer patients towards decisions they feel they should make, rather than grasp the nettle of the rather more complicated shared decision-making process. In particular, the finding that at least one doctor would steer the patient away from options for the doctor's own ends is very important, as it is possible that it is more widespread, just rarely admitted to.

The difficulty is, as we have seen, that different people will be happy with different levels of risk. The 'risk' health professionals run if we make decisions on behalf of patients is that we might not match their level of understanding or acceptance. We may feel that we have read the evidence, done the thinking and made a decision – but that decision may not have been made in the context of that specific patient. As we saw in Chapter 1, risks that people are prepared to take depend on their own values or belief systems. Additional complications such as framing effects and biases, such as availability or confirmatory bias, also affect patients, resulting in the difference between objective risk and perceived risk.

Patients talking

We can understand more about the 'risks' of poor communication if we take time also to hear the patients' perspectives. The difficulties when doctors do not take the time to explore, or when they incompletely understand, the patient's perspective are illustrated by this patient who wrote to her local evening paper:

'I am 37 and three months pregnant. My doctor is insisting that I have an amniocentesis test. However, I have heard that there is a risk that this can induce a miscarriage ... my doctor thinks this risk is negligible when set against the possibility of someone my age having a child with Down's syndrome. ... I would never dream of having a termination even if the baby did have a disability, so why is my doctor still putting pressure on me? I was so happy when I learned I was pregnant again, but the worry of all this is making me wish I wasn't.'

A similar scenario is recounted here:

'When I said I didn't want the AFP (alpha fetoprotein) test to see if it was Down's, they [the doctors] looked at me like I was mad. I think they thought I didn't know what I was talking about so they just started to repeat all the stuff about my age and the risk. I could have told them that I wasn't going to have a termination even if it was positive so they could have saved their breath. But they just assumed I didn't understand.'

There is often a gap between what doctors and other health professionals say and what is heard by patients. A reliable risk communication tool must take this into account. At times of anxiety or apprehension, patients need clear explanations but also to feel that the doctor understands what it is like for them to be receiving the news. A balance between clear discussion and personal contact must be struck.

'I was 40 and my wife was 39 and we already had six kids – the youngest then was eight years old. So to find my wife was pregnant was a shock out of the blue. She went to hospital for her first scan. I couldn't go with her as I was working on nights. When she came home she woke me up and she was crying her eyes out. They had told her that they thought it was Down's syndrome – the baby had a really fat neck and that's a sign of Down's syndrome. That was a Friday and they asked us to come in [to hospital] on the Monday. We'd had the weekend to think about it. Dr S came in to us and said: "Are you going to terminate or

continued overleaf

what?" He asked us as if he was saying "Do you want a loaf of bread?" or ordering a pint – as if it was something or nothing. The tone of his voice showed he was asking us a question without any thought. We were shocked, as they hadn't told my wife we had to make a decision. We were that shocked we never said anything. Then we were sent to see a counsellor that day and she told us about special schools [for people with Down's syndrome]. We had no fears we would have coped with a child with Down's syndrome – we already had one disabled son and coped with him and we knew people with Down's syndrome who were not much different to other people except what they looked like.

When doctors have been working for years they become like a butcher who is dealing with meat or like a bingo caller. They go on auto-pilot. Some lose empathy with people and should go on update courses to learn that they are talking to human beings. It happens in all professions when you've been doing it so long. You're not thinking of people as individuals – you are just working until you go home.

Luckily, thank God, there was nothing wrong with her [the baby] and we didn't terminate. They lost the blood tests and my wife was very anaemic at the end of her pregnancy. She's aged four now and a really lovely girl. It just goes to show that they don't know everything these doctors and they should act like that every now and again.'

The above quote was taken from a conversation with a taxi driver, and a second taxi driver helped reveal the extent to which patients expect to be involved in shared decision making.

'Doctors are like motor mechanics – they should involve the public in decisions – whether to replace or patch a faulty part or send for a second opinion. The majority of a motor mechanic's job is replacing faulty bits – like hospital doctors do.

If the patient keeps coming back the doctor should think there is something wrong. As a mechanic I would think there's something wrong if your car kept overheating and you kept coming back.

My doctor is really good and talks to me straight about my smoking. Good doctors tell you the truth and don't look down their noses at you and think you are illiterate.'

We can see that the language of risk is open to misunderstandings and subject to variations, or dialects, just as any language is. Work needs to be done on access to easily administered, reliable risk scales, not least because without them patients are relying on doctors who may themselves be misinterpreting risk levels. Without a clear grasp of risk information doctors may be tempted to 'make it up as they go along', either through a simple lack of information about risk level or poor understanding of relative risk.

Unless these factors are taken into account, this type of discussion of risk does not reflect true respect for autonomy. The health professional who makes decisions on behalf of patients or feels threatened when patients have access to alternative sources of information is not truly acting in partnership with patients.

Shared decision making

We can describe the current thinking on shared decision making with three models:

1 the professional model
2 the reasonable patient model
3 the subjective patient model.

In each of these models, shared decision making is made more difficult if there is lack of knowledge about facts relating to the risks. Not knowing a risk level can be worse than being overcautious. Health professionals need to observe the trust patients place in them by keeping up to date, the first step in effective risk communication.

In the 'professional model', the doctor hands over his expert understanding of the levels of risk with a directed plan of action. The test of 'professionalism' here might be that other doctors in this position would disclose the same level of information. This is less common these days and can be considered paternalistic – competent patients may be denied the opportunity to weigh up the evidence for themselves and make their own decisions. It has a role where the medical condition of the patient is rare, evidence from research is complicated or decisions need to be taken quickly. It depends on trust between doctor and patient. However, it is a role health professionals should adopt cautiously and only in very unusual circumstances.

The 'reasonable patient model' has been described in a discussion of risk disclosure in the Sidaway case.[4] The level of information disclosed should be that which a reasonable patient (or 'prudent patient' in Lord Scarman's judgement in the Sidaway case) would expect, whether the patient asks for that information or not. Doctors would have to ask themselves what a reasonable person in their patient's position would want to know and should satisfy themselves that such information was available to their patient. This might be called a protective approach for the medical profession, based on safety for the doctor rather than help for the patient. It might result in more information being thrust upon a patient than he or she would wish, or a feeling that they are being abandoned to make up their own mind.

The 'subjective patient model' expects the health professional to take into account the individual patient involved in the decision making. It is based on the understanding that different people are happy with different levels of uncertainty and depends on the ability of the doctor to tailor the information to the needs of each person. The difficulty with this is that doctors differ too. Some will be more comfortable than others to involve the patient in the decision making or to respect the decision of patients whose course of action differs from that which they would advise. It is not unknown for doctors to doubt the competence of those patients who disagree with them.

This third model relies on good communication skills and an accurate understanding of the scientific information on the part of the doctor. However, it is the model most likely to take the individual patient fully into account. The role of the doctor here could be described as 'guide' and the relationship of doctor and patient is nearest to the famous definition of them given by Julian Tudor Hart as 'co-producers of health'.

Risk scales

The literature contains several attempts to draw up tools that can increase understanding of risk. A good risk scale will enable risks to be compared and described, and will increase understanding for an individual patient about the risk he or she faces. Risk scales should lead to decision making that patients feel comfortable with. They need also to be acceptable to both the patient and the doctor.

A systematic review of the use of decision aids by patients facing treatment or screening decisions concluded that they can improve knowledge, reduce conflict at the time of decision making and stimulate patients to be more involved without increasing their anxiety.[5] Despite the variety of decisions, interventions and measuring tools that were surveyed, all the trials showed that decision aids do a better job than 'usual care' in terms of increased knowledge of options and outcomes.

As we have seen in Chapter 1, decision making will depend on a person's values and beliefs, and this study also showed that patients using a decision aid felt more comfortable with their choices and clearer with regard to personal values. This would indicate that decisions made in this way are more likely to be followed through. Patients persuaded by their doctor to take a certain course of action may well change their mind when away from the consulting room and free from pressure.

Work has also been done on doctors' perceptions of the effect that communication tools have on consultations.[6] In this study, unsurprisingly, providing doctors with information on risks and benefits of treatment options was well received and found to help communication. In particular, however, the doctors felt that a range of complementary formats for providing information about risk would be better than individual strategies. The study used verbal scales with words such as 'frequently' or 'sometimes', numerical scales, such as percentages and number-needed-to-treat, and graphical presentations of information.

So what risk scales do we already have that we could use to describe risk? The following is a brief description of the more important scales.

The Paling Perspective Scale©

Proposed by John Paling, from Oxford and now at the Environmental Institute in Florida, this scale was devised 'for when you are up to your armpits in alligators and you don't know which way to turn'.[7] This allows us to place the risks of some life events in order along a logarithmic scale. Adverse medical events can then be placed on the scale for comparison. It is useful for irreversible risks rather than reversible risks such as the adverse effect of drugs that will disappear when the drug is stopped. The scale appears (Figure 2.1) with the kind permission of John Paling. It can be downloaded from the

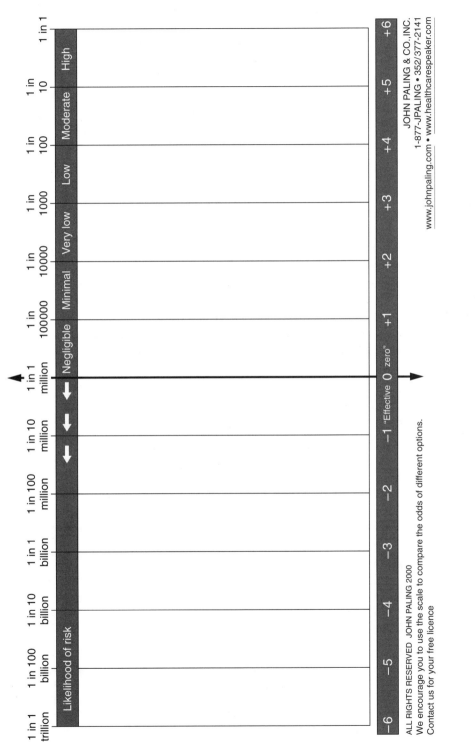

JOHN PALING & CO.,INC.
1-877-JPALING • 352/377-2141
www.johnpaling.com • www.healthcarespeaker.com

Figure 2.1: The Paling Perspective Scale© for physicians and patients. 'Helping the public put life into perspective.'

Internet at http://www.healthcarespeaker.com and users can fill in individual data to help communicate risk comparisons.

In using this scale, some authors have chosen comparators such as the risk of being a murder victim, or of being killed in a road accident or an accident at home. The main problem with these choices is that people's experience and bias about the likelihood of these events will then colour how likely they feel the adverse medical events are. The risk of winning the lottery is an obvious such 'delusional comparator' that may result in distorted appreciation of risk. As Kant said, we see things 'not as **they** are but as **we** are'.

Verbal scale

The previous Chief Medical Officer, Sir Kenneth Calman, in 1996 put forward commonly used words and suggested a numerical value for them (*see* Table 2.2). This was an attempt to standardise descriptive terms and at the same time answer the public's question as to what is meant by 'safe'. In particular, it was suggested that the use of the word 'negligible' was not to be used to imply that there is no risk or that the outcome is not important. The latter will depend on what that outcome is and will almost certainly matter to the person involved.

Table 2.2: Descriptions of risk in relation to the risk of an individual dying (D) in any one year or developing an adverse response (A)[8]

Term used	Risk range	Example	Risk estimate
High	<1:100	(A) Transmission to susceptible household contacts of measles and chickenpox	1:1–1:2
		(A) Transmission of HIV from mother to child (Europe)	1:6
		(A) Gastrointestinal effects of antibiotics	1:10–1:20
Moderate	1:100–1:1000	(D) Smoking 10 cigarettes a day	1:200
		(D) All natural causes, age 40	1:850
Low	1:1000–1:10 000	(D) All kinds of violence and poisoning	1:3300
		(D) Influenza	1:5000
		(D) Accident on road	1:8000
Very low	1:10 000–1:100 000	(D) Leukaemia	1:12 000
		(D) Playing soccer	1:25 000
		(D) Accident at home	1:26 000
		(D) Accident at work	1:43 000
		(D) Homicide	1:100 000
Minimal	1:100 000–1:1 000 000	(D) Accident on railway	1:500 000
		(A) Vaccination associated polio	1:1 000 000
Negligible	<1:1 000 000	(D) Hit by lightning	1:10 000 000
		(D) Release of radiation by nuclear power station	1:10 000 000

The author notes that this will deal only with the size of a risk and not how that risk will be perceived or managed. It cannot take into account a patient's risk–benefit gamble.

Community risk scale

A paper, again written by Professor Sir Kenneth Calman with Geoff Royston, head of operational research at the Department of Health, and published in the *BMJ* in 1997, proposed a community risk scale as a way of communicating about risk.[9] This allows discussion of risk in terms of 'You would expect this to happen to around one person in a street or one in the whole country' (*see* Figure 2.2 overleaf).

Duckworth's risk-o-meter

Statistician Frank Duckworth presented his risk-o-meter to the Royal Statistical Society in July 1999. It is logarithmic and phrased like a Richter scale, from 1 to 8 (*see* Table 2.3). It ranks events according to the likelihood that they will result in death, and Duckworth hopes it can be used to compare medical risks. He feels that people will be able to use it to compare the risks they are given with those they have experienced.

Table 2.3: Rank risk of death from different activities[10]

Event	*Score*
Imminent suicide	8
Russian roulette (one game)	7.2
Continuing to smoke:	
male aged 35 smoking 40 per day	7.1
male aged 35 smoking 20 per day	6.9
male aged 35 smoking 10 per day	6.7
Deep-sea fishing over 40 years	6.4
Rock climbing over 20 years	6.3
Accidental falls (lifetime risk for a newborn)	5.5
Lifetime car travel (newborn)	5.5
Homicide (lifetime risk for a newborn)	4.6
Rock climbing (one session)	4.2
100-mile car journey (sober, middle-aged male driver)	1.9
1000-mile flight	1.7
Death by asteroid impact (lifetime risk for a newborn)	1.6
100-mile train journey	0.3

Risk magnitude	Expect about one adverse event per	Examples: deaths in Britain per year from:
10 (1 in 1)	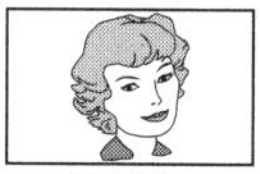 person	–
9 (1 in 10)	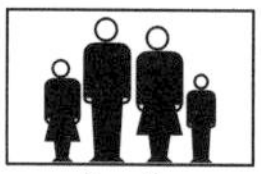 family	–
8 (1 in 100)	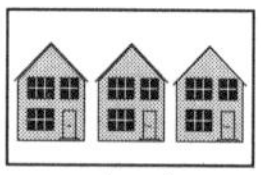 street	Any cause
7 (1 in 1 thousand)	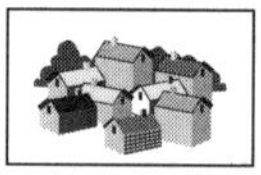 village	Any cause, age 40
6 (1 in 10 thousand)	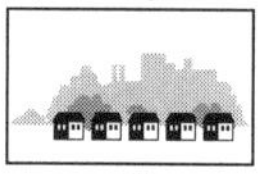 small town	Road accident
5 (1 in 100 thousand)	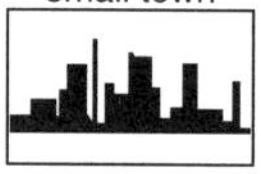 large town	Murder
4 (1 in 1 million)	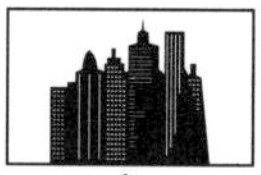 city	Oral contraceptives
3 (1 in 10 million)	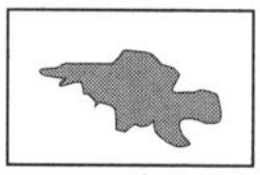 province/country	Lightning
2 (1 in 100 million)	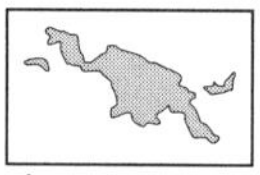 large country	Measles
1 (1 in 1 billion)	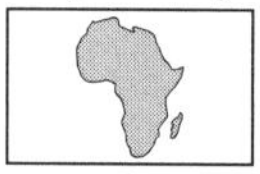 continent	–
0 (1 in 10 billion)	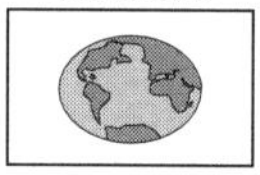 world	–

Figure 2.2:   Community risk scale. Reproduced by kind permission of Sir Kenneth Calman.

The lottery scale

An interesting suggestion was made in a letter to the *BMJ* in 1998.[11] Based on figures supplied by the lottery organisers, the authors designed a near-logarithmic scale of risk showing the probability of matching a number of balls for a £5 stake (*see* Table 2.4). A three-ball prize (£10) corresponds on this scale to a risk of between 1 in 10 and 1 in 100. Patients might be expected to have knowledge of how likely these winning events will be, which enables them to make a comparison.

Table 2.4: Probability of matching number of balls for £5 stake, compared with verbal and logarithmic scales of probability

Number of balls	Probability	Verbal scale	Logarithmic risk scale
3	1:11	High	9
4	1:206	Moderate	8
4 + bonus	1:8878	Low	7
5	1:11 098	Very low	6
5 + bonus	1:466 127	Minimal	4–5
6	1:2 796 763	Negligible	<4

Some of these scales will clearly be useful for some consultations between health professionals and patients.

A risk scale that helps us to define what is meant by numerical level of risk, such as 1 in 10 000, however, only tells half the story. As we have seen, reliable decision making about risks and benefits depends on actual knowledge of the outcomes of certain activities or interventions. A more useful risk tool will take into account that there may be a lack of information about risk level, so that comparators may not help.

One of the outcomes of the study on the perspective of doctors in training for general practice of the usefulness of risk communication tools quoted above,[6] was that doctors felt it would be helpful to have a resource pack of risk information in a variety of formats about common problems in general practice. Many of them noted that the lack of data and difficulty in keeping up with information on risk were major hindrances to communicating risks. Examples requested were using the oral contraceptive pill, the benefits and disadvantages of lipid-lowering treatments, treatment of hypertension and the risks of common operations.

We have gathered together information that may be helpful as a basis for shared decision making in The Risk Ready Reckoner (Table 2.5). It is repeated at the back of this book for ease of use.

Table 2.5: The Risk Ready Reckoner©. Facts about some common and not-so-common risks to aid in shared decision making

Risk factor (reference)	Risk estimate	Verbal scale	Comparator (in UK)
All natural causes risk of death aged 40 [4]	1 in 850	Moderate	Like one person in a village
Risk of dying in any one year from smoking 10 cigarettes per day [4]	1 in 200	Moderate	
Lifetime risk of cancer (any type) [9]	1 in 3	Very high	
Breast cancer in women [7]			
– lifetime risk	8 in 100	High	Like a three-ball win on the lottery
– baseline expected risk aged 50–75	45 in 1000	Moderate	
– on HRT for 5 years	47 in 1000	Moderate	
– on HRT for 10 years	51 in 1000	Moderate	
– on HRT for 15 years	57 in 1000	Moderate	
Osteoporosis			
– lifetime risk of a 50-year-old woman [5]	4 in 10	Very high	
– lifetime risk for men	13 in 100	High	
– risk of hip fracture if on HRT	13 in 100	High	
Cardiovascular risk			
– event in next five years for a non-smoker aged 50 [6]	47 in 100	High	
– on HRT for 5 years	36 in 100	High	
Ovarian cancer [3]			
– baseline risk aged 45	1 in 10 000	Low	Like the risk of death per year in pregnancy
– with an affected sister	5 in 100	High	
– with an affected mother	7.5 in 100	High	
Oral contraceptive pill (OCP)			
– death (non-smoker, under 35) [2]	1 in 77 000	Very low	Like the risk of being a murder victim
– thrombosis [1]	15 in 100 000	Low	Like the risk of dying in a car accident
Oral contraceptive pill (OCP) (cont)			
– baseline risk of thrombosis (not on pill) [1]	5 in 100 000	Very low	Like the risk of a man dying in a soccer accident
– thrombosis on third generation OCP [2]	30 in 100 000	Low	Like death from any kind of violence or poisoning
– breast cancer aged 45 with 5 years on OCP [10]	11.1 in 1000	Moderate	
– baseline risk aged 45 with no OCP use [10]	10 in 1000	Moderate	
Pregnancy in the UK [8]			
– death from all causes	1 in 10 000	Low	Like one in a small town
– deep venous thrombosis [1]	60 in 100 000	Low	
– miscarriage	1 in 4	Very high	
– congenital abnormality	2 in 100 births	High	

continued opposite

Table 2.5: Continued

Risk factor (reference)	Risk estimate	Verbal scale	Comparator (in UK)
Amniocentesis [8]			
– discovery of an abnormality	1 in 600 tests	Moderate	The risk of death per year for hang gliders
– miscarriage	1 in 100	Moderate	Like the risk of dying from smoking 15 cigarettes per day
Risks of other medical intervention			
– contracting HIV infection from donated blood	1 in 2 500 000	Negligible	Like a six-ball win (jackpot) on the lottery
– contracting hepatitis C from donated blood	1 in 300 000	Minimal	Like the risk of dying in a railway accident
– additional lifetime risk of fatal cancer from abdominal CT [9]	1 in 2000	Low	Like an extra 4.5 years of background radiation
– additional lifetime fatal cancer risk resulting from a chest X-ray examination [9]	1 in 1 000 000	Negligible	Like an extra three days of natural background radiation

1   *Drugs and Therapeutics Bulletin* (2000) Oral contraceptives and cardiovascular risk. **38**(1): 1–5.
2   Calman K (1996) Cancer: science and society and the communication of risk. *BMJ.* **313**: 799–802.
3   Stratton JF *et al.* (1998) A systematic review and meta-analysis of family history and risk of ovarian cancer. *Br J Obstet Gynaecol.* **105**: 493–9.
4   Henderson M (1990) *The BMA Guide to Living with Risk.* Penguin, Harmondsworth.
5   Grady D *et al.* (1992) Hormone therapy to prevent disease and prolong life in postmenopausal women. *Ann Int Med.* **117**: 1016–37.
6   Anderson KV *et al.* (1991) Cardiovascular disease risk profiles. *Am Heart J.* **121**: 203–8.
7   Collaborative Group on Hormonal Factors in Breast Cancer (1997) Breast cancer and hormone replacement therapy: collaborative reanalysis of data from 51 epidemiological studies of 52,705 women with breast cancer and 108,411 women without breast cancer. *Lancet.* **350**(9084): 1047–59.
8   Cusick W and Vintzileos AM (1999) Fetal Down's syndrome screening: a cost effectiveness analysis of alternative screening programs. *J Matern Fetal Med.* **8**(6): 243–8.
9   The Royal College of Radiologists (1998) *Making the Best Use of Department of Radiology Guidelines for Doctors* (4e). The Royal College of Radiologists, London.
10   Guillebaud J (1997) *Contraception Today* (3e). Martin Dunitz, London.

References

1   Ley P (1988) *Communicating with Patients.* Stanley Thornes, Cheltenham.

2   Seymour L, Woloshynowych M and Adams S (2000) Patient perception of the risk associated with elective heart surgery. *Healthcare Risk Resource.* **3**(1): 8–11.

3   Godfrey SE (1999) The Pap smear, automated re-screening and negligent non-disclosure. *Am J Clin Path.* **111**: 14–17.

4   Montgomery J (1997) *Healthcare Law.* Oxford University Press, New York.

5   O'Connor AM *et al.* (1999) Decision aids for patients facing health treatment or screening decisions: systematic review. *BMJ.* **319**: 731–4.

6   Edwards A, Elwyn G and Gwyn R (1999) General practice registrars' responses to the use of different risk communication tools in simulated consultations: a focus group study. *BMJ.* **319**: 749–52.

7   Paling J and Paling S (1993) *Up to Your Armpits in Alligators.* The Environmental Institute, Florida.

8   Calman K (1996) Cancer: science and society and the communication of risk. *BMJ.* **313**: 799–802.

9   Calman KC and Royston GHD (1997) Risk language and dialects. *BMJ.* **315**: 939–42.

10   Dickinson D (1999) Measuring risk on a scale of one to eight. *Patient.* **29**(1): 6.

11   Barclay P *et al.* (1998) Lottery can be used to show risk. *BMJ.* **316**: 1243 (letter).

PART TWO

Clinical risk management

CHAPTER THREE

Changing the culture

If we practise risk management in primary care settings we should be able to analyse and then reduce risks to make our healthcare services safer and more effective.

Where are we now?

Communicating and managing risks with individual patients is very much about finding ways to explain risks and elicit people's values and preferences so that all these dimensions can be incorporated into the decisions they make. When this was covered in Chapters 1 and 2 the focus was as much on helping individuals to assess outcomes (e.g. treatment of cancer) as with grappling with the probabilities.

Risk management at a practice level, on the other hand, centres mainly on 'facts' rather than 'values' or 'preferences'. Facts such as the probability that a hazard will give rise to harm – how bad is that risk, how likely is it, when will the risk happen if ever and how certain are we of our estimates about the risks? This applies just as much whether the risk is an environmental or organisational risk in the practice, or a clinical risk.

Risk assessment establishes actual levels of risk. It should lead to action to prevent or control those risks to people or the organisation or business that otherwise might be affected. Risk assessment entails the scientific assessment of the size and nature of a risk, which is followed by a decision on whether to:

- transfer the risk
- negate the risk
- share the risk
- ignore the risk
- accept the risk.

The type of action or inaction we choose to take will depend on the probability of the risk occurring or recurring, the impact of the risk if it should occur and the costs of preventing or avoiding the risk.

> Essentially we need to decide: how safe is safe enough?

The four stages in risk management[1] are to:

- identify the key risks and any triggers, encouraging staff to volunteer and discuss observed risks and adverse events
- analyse the risk – how common is it, are there patterns or trends, what impact does it have, does that impact matter? And investigate high-risk occurrences
- control the risk – what we can do about it. And implement changes in practice as necessary, and feed back to staff
- cost the risk – look at the cost of getting it right versus the cost of a risky outcome.

Risks occur whether or not we introduce a new intervention. If we do, then there are the risks that people may forget or ignore what the new system or procedure is, or be unaware of it if communication is poor or non-existent. If we do not introduce a new intervention, we may be in danger of perpetuating outdated practices or not being sufficiently flexible to meet new or rising demands.

Sometimes managing or controlling one risk has the knock-on effect of creating new or greater risks elsewhere. If we do not have a grasp of the bigger picture, we can make things worse – and more risky. For instance, if we sprinkle salt on the path leading up to the surgery when it is icy to reduce the risk of patients falling down, we increase our risk of being held financially liable for someone actually slipping down; if we treat someone's joint pains with an anti-inflammatory drug, we increase their risk of a stomach ulcer.

A baseline assessment of the extent of risk management being undertaken by the 23 practices in one PCG in the West Midlands found that:

- 22 practices had a complaints system
- 20 practices reported that they learnt lessons from every complaint received
- 13 practices currently had a system in place for assessing clinical or non-clinical risks aimed at avoiding adverse outcomes
- only 8 practices had ever carried out a significant event audit or critical event analysis.

Clinical risk and clinical governance

Managing and communicating risks is integral to clinical governance, whether at an individual patient level or at an organisational level. Clinical governance 'is doing anything and everything required to maximise quality'.[1] It is about finding ways to 'implement care that works in an environment in which clinical effectiveness can flourish by establishing a facilitatory culture'.[2]

> **managing and communicating risks**
> is a core component of any
> **individual personal development plans**
> that will feed into a
> **workplace or practice personal and professional development plan**
> that is integral to the
> **workplace or practice clinical governance action plan**
> that will feed into
> **the PCG/T's or trust's business plan underpinned**
> **by the clinical governance programme**[3-5]

We have identified the following 14 themes as core components of professional and service development, which, taken together, constitute *clinical governance*.[3] All of these are pertinent to risk management in that each creates risky situations if best clinical practice is breached, staff underperform or practice systems are inadequate. These are:

- learning culture: in your practice, the PCG/T, the trust and the NHS at large
- research and development culture: throughout the NHS
- reliable data: in your practice or trust, PCG/T, the NHS as a seamless whole
- well-managed resources and services, as individuals, as a team, as a practice, across the NHS, and in conjunction with social care and local authorities
- coherent team: well-integrated teams within your practice or trust or PCG/T
- meaningful involvement of patients and the public: in your practice, PCG/T and the NHS
- health gain: activities to improve the health of patients served by your practice and through different geographical areas of the NHS
- confidentiality: of information in consultations, in medical notes, between practitioners
- evidence-based practice and policy: applying it in practice, in the PCG/T, across the trust or the NHS
- accountability and performance: for standards, performance of individuals, the practice or trust, the PCG/T and the NHS – to the public and those in authority
- core requirements: good fit between skill-mix and competence, communication, workforce numbers, morale in general practices and across the PCG/T
- health promotion: for patients, the public – targeting those with most needs
- audit and evaluation: when making changes – of individuals' and practices' or a trust's performance, of practice or PCG/T achievements and district services
- risk management: proactive review, follow-up, risk management, risk reduction.

Risk management is central to a strong clinical governance culture where quality is considered in as wide a perspective as possible to:

- sustain quality improvements
- minimise inequalities in the health of different subgroups of the population

- reduce variations in healthcare services
- define standards
- demonstrate achievements.[3]

Minimising inequalities is at the heart of clinical governance, in relation to: variations in access, service provision or standards of care, and discrimination on the grounds of age, gender, ethnicity, sexuality, disability and so on. Inequalities of people's health may also be influenced by risky lifestyles and social determinants of health, such as poor housing, low income, transport.

Clinical risk, quality and changing the culture

The government's key priorities include: cancer, coronary heart disease, services for mentally ill people, older people and children. The intention is that services for these groups will be 'faster, fairer and more convenient'. This will require a coordinated improvement in the knowledge and skills of the workforce, ready access to team-based services, and better information to patients and the public. Effective risk management is the 'glue' that will help clinicians understand what is required in the modernised NHS to sharpen up the process of the delivery of services.

The two main approaches to improving health are by focusing on measures to improve the health of the community as a whole, or by concentrating on individuals who are at the highest risk of ill health.[3] These approaches often overlap in relation to targeting high-risk groups of people as part of a more general population-based campaign. Successful strategies to achieve health gain rely on good risk management.

Managing and communicating risk by clinicians and managers will be at the heart of the effective management of change that will be necessary to achieve the planned improvements in these key priority areas and the rest of the NHS.

1   Clinical risk management will focus on identifying and prioritising those most at risk of adverse effects of ill health if their condition is not treated effectively or managed well over the long term.
2   Organisational risk management will ensure that the systems and procedures necessary to achieve excellent clinical management are in place all of the time.
3   Good communication of risk to patients with identified clinical conditions should enhance compliance with best healthcare practice and the extent of self-care and responsibility they assume.
4   Good information about the condition and communication of risk to those who have developed the condition but have not yet been identified by the NHS should lead to those individuals presenting for diagnosis and treatment at an earlier stage.

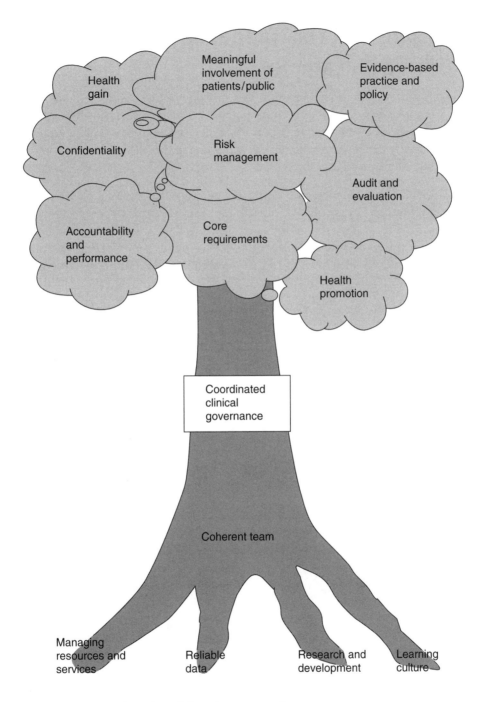

Figure 3.1:   'Routes' and branches of clinical governance.[3]

Health gain and risk management: some clinical examples

Risk factors for disease include: education, sexual behaviour, sanitation, social networks, smoking, alcohol consumption, unemployment, relative poverty, overweight, lack of physical exercise, dietary factors, occupational risks, traffic injuries, drug addiction and air pollution. Many of these are outside the influence of the NHS.

Risk management involves:

- the NHS working in partnership with non-health organisations at a strategic level and throughout the ranks
- practices, PCG/Ts and trusts having close links with local public health departments
- clinicians being aware that they are unable to influence many of the determinants of health as individuals and need to cooperate with local and national strategies.

> The continuing follow-up of civil servants in the Whitehall study demonstrates some of the differentials that exist in society with respect to health. 'After more than 25 years of follow up of civil servants aged 40 to 69 years at entry to the study, employment grade differences still exist in total mortality and for nearly all specific causes of death. The main risk factors (cholesterol, smoking, systolic blood pressure, glucose intolerance and diabetes) could only explain one third of this gradient.'[6]

There follow some examples of risk management in clinical conditions.

Depression

The potential risks for a patient in which depression is not detected and treated include: suicide, parasuicide, suffering from mental ill health and associated physical symptoms for a longer period of time, unnecessary investigations for somatic symptoms, loss of income to patient and his or her family if the wage earner is off work or dies, and poorer quality of life.

Risk management to identify and treat those with depression effectively will involve:

- education and training for GPs and staff so that they are more alert to the possibility of depression, more aware that depression may present with physical symptoms, and more familiar with best practice in length, range and type of treatments
- education and training of non-clinical staff so that they are aware of symptoms of depression and other mental health problems, and thus more tolerant of the behaviour of withdrawn or irritable patients

- heightened awareness of what are the high-risk groups for suicide: young men; frail and debilitated people, including the elderly; people who have already proposed committing suicide
- composing a disease register and following up those with depression
- tagging patient records of any vulnerable patients considered to be at high risk of any medical condition, including depression, so that any locum doctor or nurse will treat all new symptoms with great care and the receptionists will know that they should fit them in as urgent cases to be seen without question
- agreeing roles and responsibilities between everyone involved in treating depression around a practice protocol: GPs, practice nurses, community psychiatric nurses, counsellors, health visitors (especially for postnatal depression), psychologists and psychiatrists, voluntary group officers from organisations such as MIND or the Samaritans.

Diabetes

The potential risks of poorly controlled diabetes are premature death and complications, and adverse consequences from concurrent diseases.

Risk management to identify and treat those with diabetes effectively will include:

- GPs and practice staff being competent to diagnose and manage patients with all types of diabetes; for instance checking feet and eyes at least annually
- creating an effective practice organisation that has efficient systems for managing, monitoring and recalling patients with diabetes; including keeping a diabetes disease register up to date and using the register to identify and contact those who abscond from follow-up
- identifying and targeting patients at high risk of long-term complications: people who live alone, those who drink too much alcohol, those with poor eyesight, those with poor glycaemic control, those with a poor self-image, those who live in a deprived area, those with other complications of diabetes, those who smoke[7]
- individualising diabetes care, management and services to meet the needs of particular patients, with respect to cultural differences (e.g. the diet), those who are housebound, young people with frenetic lives and athletes
- motivating patients with diabetes to strive for the best possible glycaemic control; ensuring that they understand the severity, implications and risks of their condition and the potential benefits of good management.

There is some evidence that well-informed patients who actively share in making decisions about treatment have more favourable health outcomes – for instance in the improved control of the blood sugar levels in the care of diabetics.[8]

Cancer

The potential for confusing patients with explanations of risks and benefits when discussing the specificity and sensitivity of screening tests was covered in Chapter 2, which also made reference to the potential risks of adverse effects of radiation resulting from imaging investigations. And of course, the balance and nature of risks and benefits of a range of treatment and management options varies between different cancerous conditions, the expertise of the treating health professionals, the resources and equipment available, and the current health of the cancer sufferer.

Risk management will involve reducing risks to the patient as far as possible by:

- individualising the treatment and management plan according to the person – and their values, personal preferences and beliefs; explaining the risks and benefits of various options to give them an informed choice
- targeting screening programmes in such a way as to include those at most risk of the condition – including attention to the location, timing, surroundings, reminders, media information campaign
- basing all cancer treatments on the best evidence; where that is not available evaluating care and treatment or linking to larger studies that aim to provide evidence (while recruiting patients by informed consent only and with the prior approval of the local research ethics committee)
- making sure that all health professionals providing care are clear about their roles and responsibilities, especially where treatment is started by one professional and monitored at intervals, while other health professionals provide interim, everyday care
- reducing waiting times for treatment – prioritising their care in line with a clinical care pathway or other agreed protocol. Ensuring that there are no time delays when patients pass from one specialist or setting to another
- managing resources and services in the locality to ration and prioritise care such that those with cancer receive appropriate treatment and investigations as soon as possible
- setting up a local system for evaluating new anti-cancer treatments as they are launched on the market, to help other health professionals decide whether to use these new drugs in treatment.

Working in partnership with patients and the public

Meaningful involvement of users and carers and consultation with patients and public are central to the government's policy – in matching the service provided to the health needs and preferences of the population. This can only be achieved effectively if we are all speaking a common language about the risks and benefits of individuals' treatment and the health services in general. A meaningful public consultation exercise is one where information is exchanged between the NHS and those being consulted to obtain a representative opinion that feeds into the local decision-making process of the health authority, trust, PCG/T and/or the participating practices.

Involving the public in decision making about whether to accept risks or to take further action is part of the risk assessment process prior to selecting the direction of risk management. This brings into the debate all the emotions described for individual patients in Chapters 1 and 2 – voluntariness, dread, immediacy, values, beliefs and preferences – rather than the scientific facts. The scientists need to explain and interpret risk assessments, listen to the public's fears and hold open debates with the public about the acceptability of the assessed risks.

In the long-running debate in some districts over the potential fluoridation of the water supply advocated by public health experts, the scientific risk assessment is in favour of fluoridating the water to reduce the high prevalence of dental caries. This is countered by campaigners from the general public persistently promoting messages that centre on the loss of voluntariness and highlighting the dread factor – of the potential damage fluoride might have on the community's health.

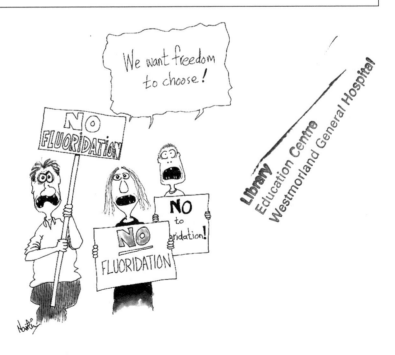

Some people use the threat of risk as a means to their own ends: they may exaggerate the potential harm that might result to encourage others to accept their leadership or ideas, or for commercial advantage. When such exaggerated claims are fed into the public arena by the media and press, the result is a bewildering array of claims and counter-claims, which confuse the public about what the health messages really are and provoke general disbelief with regard to any health messages about that topic. Confusion often arises in this way about the actual risks of various foods, such as margarine, butter and other fat spreads.

The way in which data are shared with the public influences their response. 'Perceived risk, not objective risk explains readiness to undergo screening in most models of health behaviour'. Health funding decisions are also influenced by the way data are presented; a programme predicting a 30% reduction in relative risk being perceived as more worthy of funding than the same outcome described in terms of absolute risk or numbers-needed-to-screen to avert one death from cancer. Campaigns that selectively quote incidence to 'frighten' women into undergoing mammography have been criticised.[9]

Radiation is another example of a risk that exists as a natural component of our environ-ment, but which stirs up much emotion in relation to the existence and use of nuclear power. Although the nuclear power industry has a 'safe record', public confidence is undermined by: the threat from nuclear power being imposed rather than volunteered for, the fact that there have been publicly exposed lapses in monitoring and record keeping, and fear of the impact of a significant release of radioactivity.[10]

Patient and public involvement in the planning and delivery of NHS care may occur at three levels: (i) for patients about their own care; (ii) for patients and the public about the range and quality of health services; and (iii) in planning and organising service developments.[11]

Communicating health information to the public at large

An open and accountable culture in the NHS allows sharing of information with the public about risks, costs and performance. Otherwise, consultation will be superficial and change will be unlikely in response to public opinion. The public need clear information about the health issues on which their opinion is being sought and opportunities to reflect on what they have heard before making up their minds and contributing their views, about risk for example.

Risk management will involve good communication of information to individuals or the public at large. A successful consultation exercise requires:

- commitment from the consulting organisation or healthcare unit to act on the views obtained
- unwanted results considered alongside those the consulting organisation hoped to hear
- allowing a sufficient length of time for the public consultation exercise – it takes a while to reach all subsections of a community, to engage people and gain their trust in the consultation process
- identifying funds for the consultation
- being sure of the purpose of any exercise
- obtaining a range of opinions so that the consultation is not a token activity
- working towards a change in culture where those in the NHS want to engage with people and respond to their views
- ensuring that all stages in a consultation exercise are transparent – the purpose is clear, everyone participating is well-informed, all information about the issues is brought out and there are no hidden agendas
- minimising the use of jargon, and speaking and writing any public documents in plain English, with translations for non-English speakers.

The risks of withholding information from patients are of reduced patient satisfaction and fewer opportunities for self-care. Patients ought to know what is wrong with them, what is likely to happen to them and what treatment they require. The better the information patients receive, the better able they are to participate in decision making about their own clinical management and to make informed choices about different alternatives of care. Some doctors and nurses are reluctant to share information, thinking that it may encourage patients to make more demands and so increase their workload. Others fear that parting with information may render them more vulnerable to criticism if patients are in a better position to judge health professionals' performance and the standards of treatment they receive.

Box 3.1:   Misunderstandings in prescribing decisions in general practice

Fourteen categories of misunderstandings were identified in one study. The most frequently voiced included:

- patient information unknown to the doctor
- doctor information unknown to the patient
- conflicting information
- disagreement about attribution of side effects
- failure of communication about a doctor's decision
- relationship problems.[12]

All these misunderstandings will lead to incomplete awareness of the risks involved in the choice of options for treatment and clinical management.

A variety of methods may be useful in involving users and the public in decision making about risks and benefits. Various qualitative methods may be used to gather information and views from patients, carers and the general public, such as:

- focus groups and discussion groups
- special interest patient groups: user groups, carer groups, patient participation groups, disease support groups
- general public opinion: opinion polls, citizens' juries, standing panels, public meetings, neighbourhood forums
- community development: local community development projects, healthy living centre activities
- consensus events or activities: Delphi surveys, nominal groups, consensus development conferences
- informal feedback from patients: in-house systems such as suggestion boxes and complaints.

Some methods allow interchange of views between professionals and the public – and opportunities for the public to reflect on experts' opinions before formulating their views; for example, a citizens' jury, a focus group held over two sessions with expert input to the first session (*see* Box 3.2).

Box 3.2:   Effect of discussion and deliberation on the views of focus group participants[13]

A group of patients attended two focus group meetings, two weeks apart. The participants' views about setting priorities in healthcare were systematically different at the end of their second focus group meeting compared with the beginning of the first meeting, after they had been given opportunities to discuss the issues and had time for personal reflection. About half of the participants initially wanted to give a lower priority to smokers, heavy drinkers and illicit drug users receiving healthcare, but by the end of the second meeting about one-third of these no longer wanted to discriminate against such people.

Below are some examples of methods of consultation where there are opportunities for users of the NHS or members of the public to understand and reflect on risk.

- *Focus groups*: typically last between one and two hours. Groups are usually made up of between seven and ten people. A moderator leads the group through a series of pre-prepared questions and themes, keeping the discussion constructive and focused on the topic in hand. The questions should be framed to trigger discussion about feelings and attitudes as much as knowledge or experience. The aim is to identify issues that had not previously been thought of, gain new insights about risks and the issues from the participants' perspectives, gauge the strength of feeling about different issues and spot emerging trends.

- *Citizens' juries*: inform as well as consult the members of the public participating. A typical citizens' jury has 10 to 20 people; jurors discuss and debate the issue or risks in the light of written and verbal evidence from witnesses and experts before deciding on their verdict. Biases may arise from the way in which the question is posed to the jury, the nature of the information and evidence presented to the jurors, and the identities of the witnesses, interested parties and 'stakeholders' who attend. Jurors are recruited to reflect the profile of the population in question.
- *Health panel*: the way they are set up varies. Sometimes members are recruited through open advertisement, others may be volunteers from selected groups with relatively recent experiences of the NHS. Panel numbers tend to range between 200 and 600; some operate only by postal surveys, while in others, additional focus groups are held in parallel with other survey work. Membership may last for up to three years.
- *Neighbourhood forums*: the organisers inform forum members about the risks or issues, supplying experts as requested by the forum, before views are formulated by forum members. Membership may include a mix of key or interested people in the locality, such as the clergy, nurses, teachers, etc.

Although different methods of patient involvement and public consultation may seem expensive when both direct and opportunity costs are considered, the real costs of *not* involving the public or patients in meaningful ways could be very high if the healthcare and services provided are not in tune with what is needed, or if patients are poorly served. The exact budget depends on the size of the exercise, how difficult it is to reach the target population, how skilled the personnel involved are or need to be, whether health professionals and others are incorporating the extra work into their daily activities, and what the consequent opportunity costs are.

References

1   Lilley R with Lambden P (1999) *Making Sense of Risk Management.* Radcliffe Medical Press, Oxford.

2   Chambers R and Wall D (2000) *Teaching Made Easy: a manual for health professionals.* Radcliffe Medical Press, Oxford.

3   Chambers R and Wakley G (2000) *Making Clinical Governance Work for You.* Radcliffe Medical Press, Oxford.

4   Wakley G, Chambers R and Field S (2000) *Continuing Professional Development in Primary Care: making it happen.* Radcliffe Medical Press, Oxford.

5   Department of Health (1998) *A First Class Service: quality in the new NHS.* Health Service Circular HSC (98)113. Department of Health, London.

6   van Rossum C, Shipley M, van de Mheen *et al.* (2000) Employment grade differences in cause specific mortality: a 25-year follow up of civil servants from the first Whitehall study. *J Epidemiol Community Health.* **54**: 178–84.

7   Fox C and MacKinnon M (1999) *Vital Diabetes*. Class Health, London.

8   Kaplan SH, Greenfield S and Ware JE (1989) Assessing the effects of physician–patient interactions on the outcomes of chronic disease. *Med Care.* S110–27.

9   Slaytor EK and Ward J (1998) How risks of breast cancer and benefits of screening are communicated to women: analysis of 58 pamphlets. *BMJ.* **317**: 263–4.

10   Darby S (1999) Radiation risks. *BMJ.* **319**: 1019–20.

11   Chambers R (2000) *Involving Patients and the Public: how to do it better*. Radcliffe Medical Press, Oxford.

12   Britten N, Stevenson F, Barry C *et al.* (2000) Misunderstandings in prescribing decisions in general practice: qualitative study. *BMJ.* **320**: 484–8.

13   Dolan P, Cookson R and Ferguson B (1999) Effect of discussion and deliberation on the public's views of priority setting in healthcare: focus group study. *BMJ.* **318**: 916–19.

CHAPTER FOUR

Managing common risks in general practice

The common areas of risk in general practice[1] are:

- out-of-date clinical practice
- lack of continuity of care and planning
- poor communication
- mistakes
- patient complaints
- financial risk: insufficient resources
- reputation of practitioner and practice
- staff morale and wellbeing
- disorganisation.

Out-of-date clinical practice

1 There is a risk that the evidence on which we base our practice and protocols becomes out of date without us realising it. New evidence is being published all the time. It may be published in the academic literature of other professions than our own.

Risk management involves:

- regularly reviewing (at least annually) the protocols in use in a PCG/T, trust or practice – their origin, whether there is new evidence to supplant older evidence
- searching for new evidence at the regular review, using a wide spectrum of electronic databases
- revising current protocols, where appropriate, in the light of new evidence, and to make them clearer or easier to understand
- including non-pharmacologically based interventions in the protocols that may be provided by others from outside the NHS (such as alternative practitioners) where there is evidence of benefit

- reviewing the extent to which team members are adhering to practice protocols; exploring the reasons why others are deviating from the protocols. Is it due to a lack of resources, lack of time, lack of knowledge or skills, little ownership of the protocols?

2   While incorporating change is essential, there may be risks from innovations to the practice or PCG/T organisation if they are poorly thought out, under-resourced or inappropriate for the setting and circumstances. The risks are of the innovation being abandoned halfway through, creating disorganisation or inefficiency or overwhelming staff.

> But innovation does offer the chance to avoid, minimise or control risks by trying out a new approach to the situation that led to the original hazards arising.

Risk management capitalises on opportunities for innovations but also involves:

- practice team discussions that consider the implications of any change before starting on the first steps of an innovation
- identifying the resources that will be necessary to see the whole innovation through until it is fully operational before starting out
- exploiting new technology where outdated equipment contributed to errors being made or where new technology will save on time and resources
- predicting the expertise and manpower that will be needed for any innovation – and planning so that any recruitment, education and training are completed by the anticipated start date of the innovation.

3   One reason for out-of-date clinical practice is that clinicians and managers are unaware of the latest research evidence or are reluctant to apply it. There is a considerable gap between research findings that 'prove' best practice, and health professionals and managers applying those findings in their everyday work, which will not be bridged without a proactive approach.

> Research and development are essential activities in the understanding of whether or not care is effective and how to make best use of resources.

So if we are to encourage the application of research-based theory into everyday practice we should:

- demonstrate the impact on patient care when we do implement lessons from research
- motivate people to tackle the change – show why the change is necessary and important, who else supports the change, how problems associated with the proposed change can be solved
- search for the evidence about best practice and incorporate it as a routine aspect of our work in the practice

- consider what individual beliefs, attitudes and knowledge influence professionals' and managers' behaviour
- identify factors likely to influence the proposed change
- target interventions at overcoming potential barriers to applying research evidence
- keep people informed by describing the evidence and need for change in words and ways they can comprehend
- set up mechanisms that encourage implementing changes in practice when substantial new research is published: for example, practice meetings where new findings can be reported, a cascade system to relay information, feedback from PCG/T about best practice based on new research.

4 The health benefits of an intervention need to be shown to be worthwhile before they are adopted on a wide scale in practice.[2]

Risk management to reduce the risks of an untried policy or clinical management being unleashed before it has been properly evaluated with unknown repercussions involves:

- linking clinical effectiveness to local needs and priorities
- keeping clinicians, managers, policy makers and patients involved in the process
- ensuring that any intervention is thought to be relevant and worthwhile from all these perspectives
- taking patients' and the public's values and beliefs into account when evaluating the risks and benefits.

Serum cholesterol is a poor screening test for ischaemic heart disease because although it is a strong risk factor for ischaemic heart disease in aetiological terms, the association is not sufficiently strong for it to be used as a good screening test.[3]

---

5 The overuse of radiological investigations puts patients at risk from unnecessary X-rays. Indirect risks arise as excessive investigations turn up other abnormalities, which in turn create further investigations that show the original abnormality to be of little consequence, and a great deal of anxiety for the patient and doctor.

All GPs live with uncertainty as part of their everyday professional lives in managing patients' illnesses. Too many referrals or investigations to eliminate all possibilities may have direct or indirect risks for the patient.

Risk management will involve:

- reducing inappropriate referrals; for instance, education and training for doctors and nurses in particular conditions where there are too many referrals for radiological investigations or of low-risk patients referred for a second opinion to a hospital consultant

- understanding how clinicians' own personality types affect our test-ordering frequency; introverts have been shown to refer and investigate significantly more often than extroverts do[4]
- establishing care pathways where practitioners involved in the whole pathway of care agree explicit referral criteria.

6 Health policies and strategies will not achieve what they set out to do if they are based on common health economic fallacies 'that are either logically wrong or not supported by the evidence'.[5] Risk management will involve thinking more deeply about all these issues rather than repeating many of these fallacies without the evidence to substantiate them. Some wrongly conceived fallacies are reported to be:[5]

- *'Advances in medical technology increase healthcare costs'*: wrong. The opposite is the case ... if a new drug or appliance does the same job at a lower cost.
- *'The ageing of the population will lead to a dramatic increase in healthcare costs'*: probably wrong ... patterns of morbidity are also changing so that the health of a person is likely to be improving with age ... costs of services is related to proximity of death more than age ... and ageing is supplying more informal carers who are fit and able to help.
- *'Buildings are expensive'*: wrong. The cost of operating services far exceeds the cost of a building that serves for 40–100 years.
- *'Better health services pay for themselves by getting people back to work'*: wrong. The relationship between health services and ability to work is slight, both because only a small proportion of interventions increase ability to work, and because most are given to people below and above working age.
- *'Costs of care will be lowered by "rationalising" services and closing smaller hospitals'*: wrong. Evidence of economies of scale in hospital services is hard to find.
- *'We should focus resources on those diseases that are responsible for the largest burden of morbidity and premature deaths'*: wrong. To maximise the impact of health interventions we should concentrate on the size of the solutions and not the size of problems.
- *'It is better to focus health promotion on those who are young and fit'*: probably wrong. Focus on older, sicker people means that fewer interventions make more difference to more motivated people. The costs of achieving primary or secondary prevention depend on how easy it is to identify the relevant population group and how easy it is to achieve the required change.

Lack of continuity of care and planning

1 Boundaries between and within primary and secondary care sectors can prevent effective teamwork, creating risks for the patient from poorly coordinated care or inconsistent clinical management. Teamworking is essential to the vision of the future of the NHS, to provide more user-friendly, and easier access to, primary care and an increased range of healthcare services by an increasingly multidisciplinary primary care workforce.

Improving the cohesion of teams will involve:

- promoting models and describing successful examples of more integrated care
- greater integration between health and social services in relation to planning and provision of services
- pooling service and education budgets of different organisations to encourage multi-professional teamworking
- more opportunities for working together across disciplinary boundaries or organisational interfaces so that there are cultural changes as those involved learn to appreciate the benefits of teamwork.

2   There are risks of disjointed or contradictory patient care as patients cross from one setting to another if there is no agreement about the evidence for best practice across these interfaces.

Risk management will involve:

- devising clinical care pathways as an agreed, timed framework for treating the most common conditions; this will increase the 'seamlessness' of care across the primary–secondary care interface, and between members of the employed practice team and attached staff working in the community
- implementing clinical care pathways by holding educational sessions to explain and promote the pathways, and to encourage understanding of professionals' differing roles and responsibilities and how they fit together
- encouraging ownership of clinical care pathways by involving representatives of all professional and managerial interests in devising and reviewing the pathways
- thinking as widely as possible about a condition so that all organisations with an influence on the outcome of that particular medical condition contribute to drawing up and applying that pathway; for instance a clinical care pathway for people suffering from dementia will involve social workers, financial advisers, housing officers, voluntary groups, etc., as well as clinicians and managers and non-clinical staff working in the NHS.

3   The delivery of healthcare in the future will very much focus on team-based care centred on the needs of the patient. At present, many in a practice team are not aware of what others' exact roles and responsibilities are or what other professionals might contribute to the team. Multidisciplinary learning[6] is seen as essential for creating a coherent team that works well together.

The barriers to multidisciplinary learning include: isolation of health professionals even many of those who appear to work in a team; 'tribalism' as different disciplines protect their traditional roles and responsibilities; and reluctance to develop or accept new models of working and extended roles.[6]

So we need to:

- use opportunities for multiprofessional learning to bring the various professionals together to focus on topics that they all consider important
- demonstrate some tangible improvements that arise from multidisciplinary learning
- be proactive about helping various professionals in the practice team overcome fear of, and resistance to, change
- break down rigid boundaries between educational budgets to allow pooling of funds and encourage multiprofessional learning
- use one professional's expertise to teach others in the team about specific topics that will encourage mutual trust and respect among practice team members.

4   Health improvement programmes are not expected to show tangible results for many years. Projects that are only short-term or poorly evaluated may be a waste of resources when health gains require long-term, sustained programmes with agreed milestones for use in evaluation.

Avoiding the risk of cardiovascular disease will be affected by modifiable risk factors such as smoking, cholesterol levels and exercise habits of individuals, as well as being related to their genetic predisposition and socioeconomic status.

Testing out interventions to be sure that they are effective will involve:

- sustaining interventions long-term. For instance, HIV campaigns for safe sex were initially successful but their effects wore off unless constantly reinforced[7]
- using proxy indicators of improvement to evaluate healthcare and people's health, which everyone agrees are relevant to real health gains for the population
- revising health improvement programmes in the light of the interim evaluations and new evidence
- partnership working and coordination between organisations
- targeting work at minimising inequalities in people's health and healthcare
- incorporating workforce planning around health improvement programmes to anticipate workforce needs.

Poor communication

1   The risks of inadequate communication between members of the same practice team, or between individual members of the practice team and others from outside the practice – in the PCG/T, a local trust or the health authority, or between practitioners or practice staff and patients – are that messages and guidance are not passed on creating chaos and disorganisation.

Risk management will include:

- communicating the same information at various times to everyone in the practice team, especially those who work shifts or usually work away from the main premises, for example in a branch surgery
- communicating in the right way: use direct communication whenever possible, keeping the message short and simple; communicate at the right time (usually early on); be clear about what we want to communicate; seek feedback; be open and honest; and use every opportunity for communication
- being flexible and creative if there are difficulties in communication; for example having a practice policy on good communication with people who are deaf or visually impaired.

In a review of four clinical trials, 'better health', measured physiologically (blood pressure or blood sugar), behaviourally (functional status) or more subjectively (overall health status), was consistently related to positive aspects of doctor–patient communication.[8]

---

2 Good communication is one of the key characteristics of a well-functioning team. Others are: clear team goals and objectives, and clear lines of accountability and authority, with specific individual roles for team members.

The aspects of good communication that should be nurtured for a coherent team include:

- good leadership based on democracy
- encouraging full participation by team members
- confronting conflict when it arises
- monitoring team objectives
- giving feedback to individuals and on the team performance in general
- celebrating external recognition of the team
- rewarding members of the team in appropriate ways; for example recognition of good work done, more responsibility
- arranging in-work and out-of-work activities that encourage teamwork; for example an in-house project, or social and leisure activities
- meeting regularly as a practice team; and in other meetings of subteams, such as nurse teams or other clinical teams
- practical methods of regular communication, for instance via a practice newsletter.

3 If health professionals do not understand how to motivate people to change they will fail to persuade patients to desist from risky lifestyles. They need good communication techniques as well as a good understanding of how to encourage patients to listen to, and act on, key health promotion messages.

Risk management to increase patients' motivation to beat their own lifestyle risks includes:

- offering brief behavioural counselling by practice nurses[9]
- sustaining support in reduction of risk factor(s)
- calculating an individual risk for patients of dying, with and without the modifiable risk factor; and the benefit of adding any medication (for example statin drugs). Relaying information in a clear way to distinguish between relative and absolute risks. Using risk tables and charts (*see* Chapter 2)
- teaching doctors and staff about the motivational cycle and the need to work through the state of being 'ready to change' before expecting patients to be sufficiently motivated to take action and sustain that change
- distributing appropriate patient literature and advice aids to back up the key messages
- GP staff working with others in the community who are disseminating similar health messages about lifestyle risks: community development workers, health promotion facilitators, anti-poverty officers working with local government departments.

Training GPs in communication skills to instruct patients in information seeking may be a cost-effective method of increasing compliance and improving the overall health of patients.[10]

---

4 Health promotion should be individualised to the target group. The approach used for elderly people may be inappropriate for young people, who may just 'switch off' from the health messages. Young people may have different values and preferences from health professionals, and may reject sensible advice about contraception, so resulting in unintended pregnancies.

Risk management involves targeting particular groups in the most effective ways; for example targeting young people involves:

- finding out from young people how they like to be approached
- training reception staff to be flexible in dealing with young people, who may be embarrassed or shy when they visit the surgery or unaware of the practice systems
- arranging our services so that they are young person-friendly – in relation to timing, personnel, etc. For example, holding a young person's clinic that deals with contraception and lifestyle advice and help after school hours at a time when young people can drop in without being cross-questioned by their parents. Identify young people from the age–sex register and send them each a letter informing them of the new service
- advertising the practice code of confidentiality for all patients, with information especially couched to include young people
- explaining risks and benefits of interventions (for example contraception) in clear and simple language without seeming to be patronising. Being able to pitch our explanations to accommodate young people's different educational backgrounds

- looking for innovative ways to reach young people with health messages; for example, working closely with schools on projects such as peer mentors (health professionals may help teach young mentors), school nurse drop-in clinic at the general practice surgery, videos for young people by young people
- linking closely with others who are working with young people in the community to improve their lifestyles: youth group leaders, community development officers, Sure Start and other Social Services schemes, churches
- explaining effectiveness of different types of contraception in relation to conception rates and sexual diseases; and to common but reversible adverse effects or harms (altered cycling, mood swings, weight gain) and irreversible harm (heart disease, cancer).

Young adults (younger than age 30 years) were among the groups of patients least likely to participate in decision making when consulting their doctors in one study.[11]

5   Good communication is as much about being careful with whom you communicate as what you communicate. The practice code of confidentiality may be assumed rather than being explicitly stated and reinforced, so that unacceptable breaches of confidentiality could occur, particularly when staff are caught off guard when under time pressures. Doctors and staff working for the NHS must not 'use or disclose any confidential information obtained in the course of their clinical work other than for the clinical care of the patient to whom that information relates'.[12]

Risk management involves guarding against untoward breaches of confidentiality by:

- making sure that staff are fully aware of their duty of confidentiality and security of any information obtained in the course of the patient's relationship or contact with health professionals or others in the practice team
- having a protocol about when it is permissible to assume implied consent and share information with relatives. For example, sharing of information with relatives is commonly the case with terminally ill patients, but would seldom be appropriate for issues relating to reproduction
- including a clause about retaining patient confidentiality in staff contracts, so that it is clear that staff directly employed by the NHS may be subjected to disciplinary proceedings following a breach of confidentiality
- ensuring that doctors and staff are aware of the exceptions to absolute confidentiality of patients' details: such as (i) if the patient consents to others having access to their records; (ii) if it is in the public interest that personal information is disclosed, as when someone else would be placed at risk of death or serious harm (for example when a person who has uncontrolled epilepsy persists in driving a car, or as the known sexual partner of someone with HIV). A doctor should always try to persuade such patients to disclose information voluntarily to the other person who is in danger, and if they refuse warn them of the impending breach of confidentiality; (iii) if it is in the person's own interest, such as when they may be a real danger to themselves (for example being suicidal or psychotic).

6 Health professionals who are unfamiliar with the meaning of 'Gillick competent'[13] and subsequent national guidance[14] may not make every effort to persuade child patients to involve their parents as they should, or might disclose information to the parents against the child's wishes, acting against the best interests of the child.

Risk management in relation to issues of confidentiality in respect of children will involve:

- being sure that everyone in the practice team is familiar with guidance on confidentiality when supplying contraception to under 16-year olds without the knowledge of their parents or carer[14]
- being aware that the mother's consent is needed before disclosing information to the father, where the parents were unmarried at the time of the child's birth, unless he has been given parental responsibility
- knowing who has parental authority for a child who is in the residential care of the local authority and therefore to whom medical information about the child can be disclosed – to the local authority if there is a care order, to the parent if residential care is voluntary or the court has awarded responsibility to the parent
- clarifying the procedure and reminding practitioners who suspect child abuse to report their suspicions to the appropriate authority, such as social services or the police.

7 People without a 'need to know' may be able to look at patients' records and breach the practice code of confidentiality if access arrangements to notes are insecure or confused. The Caldicott rules[15] are explicit about this – *see* the box below.

The Caldicott[15] committee report has described principles of good practice to safeguard patients' confidentiality when information is being used for non-clinical purposes:

- justify the purpose
- do not use patient-identifiable information unless it is absolutely necessary
- use the minimum necessary patient-identifiable information
- access to patient-identifiable information should be on a strict need-to-know basis
- everyone with access to patient-identifiable information should be aware of their responsibilities.

Risk management to avoid breaches of confidentiality will involve:

- preventing security procedures being circumvented, including when a colleague who is the subject of a complaint applies for access to the relevant medical records which he or she is not entitled to see in a professional capacity
- communicating the practice code about access to all health staff – as they are inducted when newly appointed
- regular reminders to staff about their obligation to preserve confidentiality
- being clear about how information in patients' medical records will be anonymised if it is being used for audit that involves others from outside the practice helping with data collection or sharing the results. Where it remains possible for patients to be

identified, their informed consent should be sought prior to the audit being carried out and they should be given the opportunity to withhold consent without prejudicing their entitlement to healthcare

- if information about patients is being gathered as part of a research study, the research protocol should first be approved by the local research ethics committee.

Mistakes

1   Mistakes and omissions will continue to occur if we do not establish a positive culture of openness throughout the NHS. There may be even more serious consequences the next time. The team should learn from critical incidents (e.g. 'near misses'), significant events (e.g. where the adverse event actually happens, such as a current patient commits suicide or a patient is prescribed and takes the wrong drug), patients' complaints and audit – to stimulate change.

> Managing risks requires the development of clinical governance action plans, developing or adopting standards and audit tools, and agreeing an annual programme of risk assessments and clinical audit.

Risk management involves:

- recording significant events and 'near misses' in a central log to look for patterns or trends
- sharing of information about critical incidents, particularly 'near misses', in a supportive atmosphere so that everyone can learn from those events and make changes as appropriate
- everyone making changes as a result of analysing these adverse events to minimise the chances of a recurrence.

2   Good access to reliable and accurate data is vital. The risks of mistakes arising when a doctor or nurse has no information about a patient, especially when meeting them for the first time – or does not know what has gone on before or what the patient has been told – are profound.

> There are certain situations when the absence of information makes safe medical or nursing practice particularly difficult, such as when visiting elderly patients with complex medical histories, who have just come to reside in a nursing home and are poor historians; or when a patient has been discharged from hospital with little or no information for the practice, and the GP has little knowledge of what treatment and management the patient has had or needs.

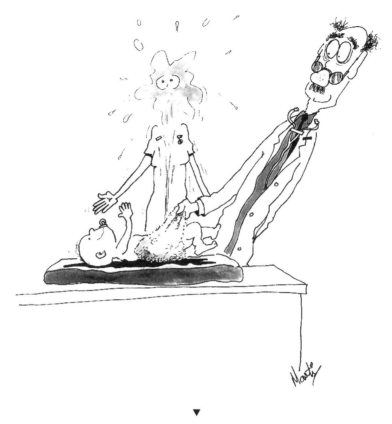

▼
Learn from your near misses

Risk management will involve:

- developing systems for access to medical records whatever the setting
- recording or retrieving information at the correct time – as soon as possible after the consultation
- working with those in other settings (e.g. secondary care if you work in primary care) to devise systems to ensure that prompt and accurate information about a patient's medical history travels with the patient – electronic 'smart' cards and shared care records have the potential to reduce these risks
- using computers to their full capacity
- establishing disease registers for diabetes, coronary heart disease, hypertension, asthma, learning disability and other priorities determined by local needs
- using the computer for entering data about all consultations
- inputting results of investigations as they arrive at the practice to reduce time wasted chasing up results when patients next consult
- setting up regular auditing of priority areas, such as review of medication
- exploiting the potential of the computer, for example in letter writing (e.g. using voice type software) and stock control of vaccinations.

A primary care team was discussing the standards of its medical records and talking about how useful record summaries were on the computer when managing patients with diabetes. It transpired during the discussion, that two of the GPs were aware of a facility for calling up the summary page of the patient's condition so that they were alerted to the presence of diabetes when monitoring that person's ischaemic heart disease, while the other three GPs did not know how to operate this function of the computer. A brief training session for the GPs, practice nurses and the practice manager on the computer by one of the knowledge-able GPs soon rectified their ignorance.

3   If those to whom tasks are delegated are not sufficiently trained or able to absorb the extra work, they make mistakes or drop the standards of care or services as a consequence. Tasks should be delegated to free up the time of the more experienced or more highly qualified clinician, but only if the person to whom the work is delegated has the time and capability to undertake the task. The current modernisation of the NHS will result in different skill-mix models of care; nurse staffing levels are often subject to skill-mix review.

Risk management to avoid problems arising from delegation should involve:

- education and training in the management of delegation for anyone who is in a position to delegate, as either an in-house or external course
- an opportunity to report back by those who have tasks delegated to them, at their annual appraisal with the practice manager for example
- anticipating changes in skill-mix and arranging education and training or recruitment of new staff prior to any changes coming into force; or arranging redundancy in a planned and supportive way if the anticipated changes will mean a scaling down of staff numbers
- practice protocols that specify the maximum responsibility allowed for particular grades of staff; lines of accountability and how that will be managed and monitored
- legible and contemporaneous note taking by all the team will allow one professional to take over care from another while being fully informed of the patient's preferences, condition, management and prognosis.

4   New members of the practice team may not be aware of a particular practice policy and their personal way of working may conflict with other members' care. We may work hard with our practice team to meet minimum standards of performance and to give a good reception to our patients. But our reputation might well be shattered by casual staff who are unaware of the practice systems and procedures – or are too rigid for our flexible ways of working.

Regularly updated and easily understood policies and guidelines will help the team members provide consistent care.

Risk management will involve:

- a good induction programme for new members to the team; appropriate induction for casual staff – for instance locum doctors should have an information pack about practice procedures and systems such as that produced by the National Association of Non-Principals
- copies of important policies, guidelines or protocols being freely available in the workplace, for example as laminated cards
- a cascade system to disseminate news and information to all the team when policies and guidelines are revised or new ones devised; this might be by electronic means, verbal feedback at practice meetings or a news bulletin board in the staff room for example
- checking the credentials and references for agency nurses or locum doctors; then senior members of the practice team should continue to supervise them.

Patient complaints

1   Traditionally, many doctors and nurses have approached their postgraduate education in an ad hoc fashion. Health professionals have attended educational events that were convenient as regards timing and location, and that interested them – rather than topics about which they needed to know more.

> Education and training should be closely tied into service development needs that relate to the needs of the local population, the government and district priorities, and the particular needs of the practice, PCG/T or hospital trust.[12,16]

So if health professionals are to provide care and services that are relevant to their patient population's health needs and personal preferences, we need to:

- redirect education and training so that it is relevant to service needs
- identify local priorities of the population through health needs assessments and by gaining input from patients and the general public to the planning and delivery of our healthcare services
- extrapolate how national and district priorities apply to us in our practices; for example the various National Service Frameworks (NSFs) for mental healthcare, coronary heart disease and diabetes, or cancer guidelines
- realign the practice personal and professional development plan with the practice business plan to arrange that everyone in our practice team addresses particular practice needs.

2   There is a risk of a patient complaint or claim for damages if a patient has not had all relevant information about a proposed procedure, and an opportunity to hear about all the 'risks' and 'benefits' that relate to their individual circumstances. A complaint is more likely if an adverse event occurs during the procedure. Informed consent requires knowing all the facts and the risks about the treatment or procedure.

Reducing the risk of a patient complaint involves:

* education and training for practitioners about the requirements for informed consent, and good ways to communicate risks and benefits (as in Chapter 2)
* consent forms that use clear and simple language and are readily to hand in all consulting and treatment rooms in the practice or NHS unit.

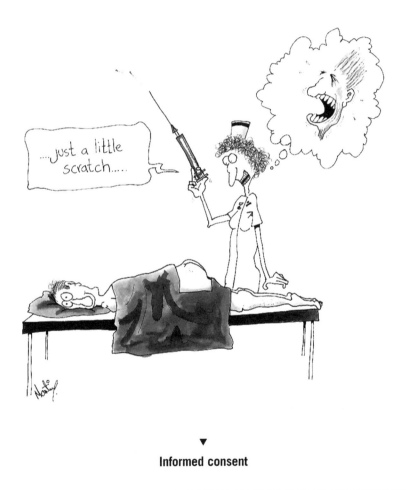

▼

Informed consent

Contextualising and personalising risk is an important part of the informed consent process.[17] A study that identified factors affecting the decisions of pregnant women to withhold their consent to participate in a clinical trial, found such conflicts of interests as a pregnant woman's protective duty to the fetus and being a good 'citizen'.

3   There are risks when patients are not involved in decision making that they will be unhappy with a particular treatment or management prescribed, because it does not fit with their values, beliefs or preferences; they may abscond from treatment and fare less well than they might have done with other alternative regimens.

The various models of decision making include:

* professional choice (paternalistic): clinician decides, patient consents
* professional as agent: clinician elicits patients' views and makes decision
* shared decision making: patient and clinician work together to negotiate an agreement
* consumerist: clinician informs, patient makes decision.

Before we can enter into shared decision making with patients we need to be in a position to understand: (i) the patient's problems: the nature and aetiology, the effects of the problem and the patient's personal circumstances; and (ii) the patient's perspective: their ideas about the problem and its management, preferences for information, relevant values and beliefs, and preferences for involvement in decision making.

Risk management will involve health professionals relaying information so that patients can:

* understand what type(s) of treatment they are being offered or prescribed and why there are these options
* understand what the risks and benefits are likely to be for them as an individual
* understand what the side effects might be
* understand the implications for the future if they do or do not accept treatment
* participate in making decisions about: which (if any) treatment to try, whether to switch treatments, whether to embark on further investigations (with what aim), whether to stop treatment or investigations, whether to consult another health professional for a second opinion or further advice
* know where to seek further information.

Then negotiate and come to a decision, checking again that the patient is in agreement before planning how to implement that decision.

In one study,[18] 71 patients who had been counselled about the different risks of reducing the long-term risk of stroke and provoking an immediate embolic stroke prior to carotid endarterectomy, were questioned one month later to assess their understanding of the risks associated with the different treatment alternatives and ability to recall the risk of suffering a stroke with each of the treatment options. Patients consistently failed to recall their risk of stroke; most remembered that surgery reduced their long-term risk of stroke; 10% overestimated the risk of surgery provoking a stroke by at least ten times; and some thought that there had been no risk of stroke from the surgery. The authors of the study recommended that 'informed consent based on verbal information alone is not enough, and that an information letter should be given to each patient as part of the process of informed consent'.

Financial risk: insufficient resources

1   There is a risk to the viability of the GP's business and the practice organisation from a drop in overall income.

Managing risks in relation to the financial side of a practice business involves:

- being aware of any additional funds for developments or practice improvements – and making well-justified applications
- keeping careful records of incomings and outgoings in close liaison with the practice accountant; keeping the records in such a way as to minimise accountants' fees
- containing the time and extent that GPs and staff work outside the practice without sufficient recompense for locum arrangements
- considering change to more cost-effective working – with new skill-mix models, a higher proportion of less-qualified staff, taking advantage of new technologies, new employment arrangements such as Personal Medical Services (PMS) pilots.

2   There is a risk to the sustained quality of healthcare and services if demand is not contained. Demand management is 'the process of identifying where, why and by whom demand for healthcare is made and the best methods of curtailing, coping with or creating this demand such that the most cost-effective, appropriate and equitable healthcare system is developed'.[19]

> Threats to the quality of healthcare from excessive demand can be moderated by rationing – by denying, delaying, deterring, diluting or terminating treatments.

Risk management to contain demand will involve:

- using needs assessments to develop services that improve effectiveness, while at the same time minimising inequalities
- looking for alternative ways of working that are more cost-effective, appropriate or equitable to replace traditional patterns
- prioritising healthcare and services according to need – at a practice level and across the PCG/T
- involving the public in local debates about rationing of NHS services and prioritisation of one service over another
- reviewing how we 'ration' care in our practices by undertaking audits to check that we are not unconsciously discriminating against patients on the grounds of gender, age or race.

One practice of five partners with 11 000 patients decided to meet patients' demand for appointments by each providing 208 booked appointments per week, running four surgeries per day over a 10- or 11-hour period. Demand from patients grew accordingly, so that the doctors could still not satisfy the demand for appointments. After 18 gruelling months, the GPs reverted to their previous arrangements of 168 booked appointments per partner per week.[20]

3   There are risks to the NHS from employing ways of working and medical interventions that are not cost-effective. A cost-effective intervention is one that gives a better or equivalent benefit from the intervention in question for lower or equivalent cost, or where the relative improvement in outcome is higher than the relative difference in cost. In other words, being cost-effective means having the best outcomes for the least input. Using the term 'cost-effective' implies that we have considered potential alternatives.[21]

An intervention must first be considered *clinically* effective to warrant investigation into its potential to be *cost*-effective. Evidence-based practice must incorporate clinical judgement. We have to interpret the evidence when it comes to applying it to individual patients, whether it be evidence about clinical effectiveness or cost-effectiveness.

Cost-effectiveness is a measure of efficiency and suggests that costs have been related to effectiveness.

Managing the financial risk involves:

* confirming that the medical intervention is clinically effective first
* comparing the alternative treatment or intervention directly with the next best treatment or intervention
* being efficient; that is, obtaining the most quality from the least expenditure, or the required level of quality for the least expenditure.

Careful attention to the quantities of drugs prescribed and cost-effective choice of drugs in repeat prescribing in one PCG freed up £128 000 in 1999–2000 to invest in additional hospital services.[19]

The cost of an osteoporotic fracture has been estimated to be £4326 per fracture, with a range from £12 254 for a hip fracture to £468 for a wrist fracture.[22] The overall cost of osteoporotic fractures to the NHS is around £950 million per year. It should be possible to work out the cost-effectiveness to the NHS of drugs that are licensed to treat osteoporosis by

continued opposite

studies demonstrating the percentage reduction in fracture rates as the number of fractures saved per year multiplied by the cost of each fracture. There will be other costs and savings to take into account according to the risks and benefits of treatments – with respect to side effects, mobility, independence, wage earning, etc. One author concluded that: 'fractures can be prevented at modest cost for groups of people at high risk ... readily available clinical risk factors such as low body weight or previous fracture can be easily used to target treatments and thus reduce the burden of fractures in the community.[23]

Reputation of practitioner and practice

1 Providing substandard care because of having faulty or unsafe equipment would soon give practices a bad reputation. Investment in equipment should keep up with best practice in clinical management protocols, so that the practice has the wherewithal to undertake appropriate investigations; for instance it is becoming more commonplace and expected that a practice will have an electrocardiograph machine (ECG) for assessing acute events secondary to ischaemic heart disease or a spirometer to assess those with chronic obstructive airways disease (COAD).

> All equipment necessary for best practice should be available and serviced regularly to provide high-quality primary care.

Ensuring the existence of effective functioning of equipment will involve:

- reviewing practice protocols for the clinical management of common conditions, and new national recommendations such as those emanating from the National Institute for Clinical Excellence (NICE) to determine whether the practice should be investing in new investigatory equipment
- reviewing legal requirements, for instance new legislation in health and safety issues, to ensure that appropriate equipment is in place and being used correctly; for instance ergonomically designed work desks and chairs for those operating visual display units (VDUs)
- checking that nebulisers, the defibrillator, the spirometer and sphygmomanometers in the practice are in good working order
- making sure that staff are competent to operate any equipment and organising training if not; for example an ECG machine is available in the practice and the practice nurse can operate it.

2 There is a potential risk of an allegation of sexual impropriety in any consultation where the clinician and patient are out of earshot and not overlooked. Some patients may find the offer of a chaperone offensive if they think it implies a lack of trust in them by the doctor. Although it is usual to consider using a chaperone when a female patient is being examined by a male doctor, male patients might also accuse female doctors of improper conduct.

Risk management to avoid allegations of sexual assault should include:

- helping staff to realise the potential risks of conducting intimate examinations without a chaperone – breast as well as genital examinations
- training members of staff who act as chaperones how to be a discreet presence in the consultation
- ensuring that there are sufficient staffing levels to allow the availability of a chaperone
- not insisting on the presence of a chaperone if the presence of a third party would restrict the patient from articulating their fears and concerns while being examined
- a well advertised in-house complaints procedure and reassurance for patients that any allegation of impropriety will be taken seriously and thoroughly investigated.

Guidance about the presence of chaperones issued by the Faculty of Family Planning and Reproductive Healthcare[24] states that:

- all clients should be advised that they may ask for a chaperone to be present
- the healthcare professional must believe that the intimate examination is necessary and will assist with the patient's care
- if a trainee is to undertake the examination he or she will be supervised
- the client must be treated with dignity and respect
- an interpreter or advocate will be present if requested
- verbal consent must have been given (to an intimate examination) after appropriate explanation.

---

3   The risk of breaching the Data Protection Act is of prosecution, which would harm a practices' reputation as well as the financial penalty imposed. The Data Protection Act (1984) requires that all personal data held on computer should be 'secure from loss or unauthorised disclosure'. Personal data is any information about someone else and includes information collected in research or interviews about named subjects. The Commissioner will need to know: name and address, a description of the data, the purpose for which the data is being held, sources from which data was/will be obtained, people to whom data may be disclosed, countries where data may be transferred and the address where subjects can obtain access to the data about themselves.

Risk management will involve:

- notifying the Data Protection Commissioner of the personal data held on computers in our workplace and the types of details we store
- reviewing the entry in the register periodically to check that it continues to provide an accurate description of our data-processing activities. If it is out of date, informing the Registrar of alterations in writing.

Further details can be obtained from the Data Protection Commissioner (tel: 01625 545745; email: mail@dataprotection.gov.uk).

The text of the Data Protection Act 1998 is at http://www.legislation.hmso.gov.uk Information about compliance with the 1998 Act is on the website: http://www.dataprotection.gov.uk

Staff morale and wellbeing

1 There is a risk to patient care if GPs and staff who are caring for them are ill or if the NHS environment is unsafe; for example there is a risk of infection to the patient through contaminated equipment or danger from noxious substances or a poor state of repair of the premises. A further risk of breaching health and safety legislation is prosecution and a hefty fine.

An employer's duty[25] with respect to the health and safety of staff and patients is to: make the workplace safe and without risks to the health of staff or visiting patients.

Risk management will involve:

- identifying hazards in the workplace: noise, potential electrical fires and infection, blood spillage, sharps
- identifying persons at risk – and in what settings; for example lone receptionists in a branch surgery
- ensuring that articles and substances are moved, stored and used safely
- providing adequate welfare facilities
- informing, instructing, training and supervising staff as necessary for their health and safety
- ensuring that equipment is safe and that safe systems of work are set and followed
- drawing up a health and safety policy statement if there are five or more employees, and making staff aware of the policy and arrangements
- providing adequate first aid facilities
- assessing the hazards and current control measures
- reducing the likelihood of hazards provoking adverse events by improving controls over them
- supporting doctors and staff after traumatic events; looking for stress hot spots and trying to minimise stress at work.

When one of the GPs in a four-partner practice developed multiple sclerosis, it took the doctor herself and the other partners many months to realise that something was physically

continued overleaf

wrong. The unwell GP had been ascribing her symptoms to her pregnancy, the medication she was taking, and the stress of combining work and home lives; she had concealed her neurological problems from her partners. She needed supportive colleagues and a safe practice environment to be able to remain at work for as long as she was fit to do so.

2   If we don't get the balance right between staffing levels and patient demand we'll have demoralised staff handing in their notice as well as the threat to maintaining the quality of healthcare we provide. Unnecessary staff turnover, excessive workload or under-usage of staff may be the result. Casual staff employed in crisis situations or to fill gaps may not fit into the team or have the same level of information about how the practice systems work.

> The quality and quantity of the workforce dictates the quality of healthcare they deliver.

So achieving a good balance between staffing levels and workload will involve:

- regularly reviewing staff numbers and posts against patients' and medical demands – to check that the balance is right in the practice team – to handle demand at specific times of the day, or of a particular nature; for instance surgery appointments for conditions patients perceive as needing 'urgent' attention
- realigning staff to meet patients' and bureaucracy demands within current resources
- new measures to contain patient demand; for instance triage by doctor or nurse, promotion of self-care and the taking of more responsibility for own health, patient education via local campaign.

3   There is a risk to anyone working in the NHS of experiencing aggression and violence from patients and their relatives. The problem of aggression and violence at work is common in the general working population, with around 35 000 people being attacked at work across the UK each year. Health professionals are at higher risk of work-related violence (including woundings, common assault, robbery and snatch theft) than the general population. Doctors and nurses are particularly vulnerable to aggression and violence: some have a great deal of daily one-to-one contact with patients who are mentally ill or disturbed, in circumstances where emotions run high and normally sane patients or relatives can suddenly become irrational or aggressive.

> Practice and community nurses, doctors and other healthcare staff who visit patients in their own homes are often unaware of the potential danger of aggression and violence being thrust upon them, because their caring nature and their role as the patients' advocate makes them relatively unsuspicious of danger.

Risk management aimed at reducing stress or fear from aggression and violence and preventing any episode occurring in the first place will involve:

- avoiding potentially dangerous situations especially when on visits to patients' homes
- staff learning how to defuse tense confrontations
- improving the workplace organisation so that the service provided is efficient and patients are less likely to become frustrated and vent their anger on you and your colleagues
- devising a workplace policy to handle a violent or aggressive incident appropriately
- equipping staff with assertiveness and anger management skills
- offering support to staff who have been victims of an attack or abuse
- learning from any violent episode and making changes to avoid a recurrence.

4   There are risks from manual handling for most clinical and non-clinical staff working in the NHS. Manual handling is an integral part of most health professionals' jobs at some time in their day. Doctors and nurses may help elderly or disabled patients up on to examination couches, district nurses may find that they unexpectedly need to lift an immobile patient when home visiting or that they have to haul equipment around, receptionists may find piles of notes heavy to carry or extract from filing cabinets whose drawers stick unless jerked.

> Besides these risks to staff, poor manual handling techniques carry an increased risk of suffering pain and distress for patients who are on the receiving end.

Risk management measures to reduce the potential risks from manual handling include:

- using an assessment tool to systematically review the practice environment and that of patients' homes for risks associated with the manual handling of patients
- purchasing a range of lifting aids according to the manual handling assessment
- replacing filing cabinets that have heavy and stiff drawers with another system of filing and note retrieval, such as open shelves at convenient heights
- buying a wheelchair as a stand-by in the practice for transporting immobile patients as necessary – if for example a patient collapses and needs to be moved to a couch or private room
- training staff in lifting techniques that are least likely to strain their backs and prevent other musculoskeletal injuries.

Box 4.1:   Hazards in the workplace[25]

For every workplace *hazard* – whether chemical, biological, physical or psychological – there is a degree of *risk*, which is the likelihood of the hazard causing harm in a particular situation. Most organs of the body can be harmed by adverse working conditions and many substances in the workplace have acute or chronic effects on health.

   A primary task of occupational health practice is to predict that risk from a knowledge of the type of hazard, the working environment and the degree of exposure (of individuals or groups) to the hazard. Having assessed the risk, occupational health and safety professionals advise employers on how to minimise it.

Disorganisation

1   Inadequate, incomplete or out-of-date medical records – paper or electronic – increase the risks of doctors and nurses making mistakes during consultations with patients, or of non-clinical staff making mistakes undertaking tasks that have been delegated to them, such as repeat prescribing, organising referrals, etc.

Risk management will involve:

* ensuring that medical records are accurate, in chronological order, summarised and up to date
* scrupulous recording of medication on paper and/or computer with review dates that are enforced
* bedding any new procedures into the everyday working of the practice team and practice systems.

2   Inconsistent data recording means that a lot of time is wasted by those who do expend effort classifying reasons for patients' consulting and entering it on computer. Incomplete practice data will underestimate the prevalence of those conditions or reasons for consultation and risk the needs of that group of patients being overlooked.

The extent to which information about patients' medical conditions and reasons for consultation is coded in a standardised way on the computer and the consistency of data entry will reduce the chances of clinicians being unaware of patients' medical risks – such as from concurrent diseases or known adverse reactions to drugs.

To improve the consistency of data recording we should:

* agree to enter or retrieve information in a standardised manner
* train staff in a standard classification system such as Read coding

- encourage all the constituent practices of a PCG/T to adopt particular Read codes so that information about morbidity and consultations can be collected on a PCG/T or district-wide basis to inform planning of services
- incorporate audit in checking whether doctors and staff are being consistent about classifying and entering data for every consultation or patient contact
- take a regular back-up of the data on the computer; storing the back-up disk off the premises in case of fire or vandalism.

A practice manager undertook an audit to identify numbers of patients classified as having angina, prior to setting up a coronary heart disease register. She found that there were only four patients classified as suffering from angina. When she looked into it she found that the GPs rarely recorded the reasons for patients consulting, usually just noting that the patients *had* consulted. The practice nurses were much more likely to use the agreed Read codes to input data about patients into the computer at every consultation. When the GPs were confronted with the evidence, they explained that they did not have time to make full records of the consultation on the computer as a routine. Appointment times were changed as a consequence, and a re-audit six months later showed that the practice had many more patients suffering from angina and the GPs had all developed the habit of entering data on the computer (with continuous nagging from the practice manager!).

---

3 Variations in practice between practitioners or between different practices, may go unnoticed and unchecked if health professionals and managers do not have the knowledge or skills to practise audit, or the motivation to review their performance in a systematic way. Although audit has been promoted and encouraged in the NHS for the past ten years, it is still not practised in a systematic way, and some health professionals still lack knowledge and skills.

Risk management will involve:

- repeated education and training of GPs and all practice staff, including the practice manager and non-clinical support staff who all have their part to play
- completing the audit cycle after review of performance and making changes as appropriate that become part of the practice's way of working
- optimising the capability of our computer system; setting it up for routine searches of patient data
- reviewing audits of our priority areas each year: for instance those identified as priority health needs for our patient population, against the standards laid out in the NSFs or from recommendations from NICE.

4 Audit may not be targeted at a problem in the right way to result in the most effective change. It is sometimes easier to audit structures (e.g. premises, records, workforce characteristics) and processes (e.g. practice procedures, medical interventions) than outcomes (e.g. impact of care or services).

Risk management to gain the maximum impact from audit will involve:

- a clear patient focus in the direction of clinical audit
- inclusion of a multiprofessional perspective
- targeting audit at the whole clinical pathway, assessing performance of the structure, process and outcome
- auditing across primary, secondary and continuing care boundaries
- linking with education and professional development.

One example that illustrates the potential benefits of applying audit in a systematic way, focusing on patient-centred outcomes, is of general practice detection and prevention of elder abuse amongst their patients.[26] The strongest factor predicting GP diagnosis of abuse was knowledge of five or more risk situations to which elderly people were exposed. The risk situations for physical abuse, psychological abuse and neglect include those of a person:

- with dementia who is left alone all day or is violent towards a carer
- who is living in a household where too much alcohol is drunk or where an adult has severe personality problems
- with a long history of domestic violence either as victim or perpetrator
- with bruising that is not satisfactorily explained
- with a paid carer who is aggressive towards the elderly person
- who repeatedly turns up at accident and emergency departments without GP involvement.

---

5   Evaluation sets out measurable targets and timescales that are realistic for the particular context and problems of the population group for whom a new service(s) or project is intended. Short-, medium- and longer-term outcomes are agreed by all the 'stakeholders' at the beginning of the project. There are risks that other factors may crop up that are not under your control and that the outcomes you originally expected, if your intervention or project worked well, are no longer viable or possible.

The regular use of evaluation should ensure that the work we do or interventions we adopt are appropriate and relevant to our patient population and will involve:

- always incorporating evaluation into our everyday work to become more practised and expert at it; using internal review undertaken by members of the team themselves
- agreeing predetermined criteria of achievement for our project or intervention
- inviting external review: evaluation undertaken by an independent person, or at least comparing what we achieve against external standards
- peer review: by peers in our field, such as others from neighbouring practices or within the PCG/T
- assessing the performance or achievement of one or more: activity, personnel, provision of service, organisational structure, objectives.

6   The risks of members of the primary care team not being clear about who does what in disease management at a practice level are that some patients may be forgotten, while others are confused by more than one member of the team managing the same part of their condition.

> A health visitor, GP and practice nurse may all advise a new mother about immunisations for the baby, but none of them may counsel her about her long-standing asthma, which is poorly controlled at night, or on exercise.

Risk management will involve:

* clarifying roles and responsibilities in any teamwork
* defining who and how each team member is appraised
* discussing audit results as a team and reviewing performance for a particular disease management, looking for ways to improve effective working
* maximising staff strengths and giving opportunities for professional fulfilment.

> A system approach to reducing errors works better than focusing on individuals. 'This approach concentrates on the conditions under which individuals work and tries to build defences to avert errors or mitigate their effects'.[27]

References

1   Lilley R with Lambden P (1999) *Making Sense of Risk Management.* Radcliffe Medical Press, Oxford.

2   NHS Executive (1996) *Promoting Clinical Effectiveness.* NHS Executive, London.

3   Wald NJ, Hackshaw AK and Frost CD (1999) When can a risk factor be used as a worthwhile screening test? *BMJ.* **319**: 1562–5.

4   Ornstein SM, Markert GP, Johnson AH *et al.* (1988) The effect of physician personality on laboratory test ordering for hypertensive patients. *Med Care.* **26**(6): 543–63.

5   Normand C (1998) Ten popular health economic fallacies. *J Public Health Med.* **20**(2): 129–32.

6   Chief Nursing Officer (1998) *Integrating Theory and Practice in Nursing.* NHS Executive, London.

7   Nardone A, Mercey DE and Johnson AM (1997) Surveillance of sexual behaviour among homosexual men in central London health authority. *Genitourin Med.* **73**: 198–202.

8   Kaplan S, Greenfield S and Ware J (1989) Assessing the effects of physician–patient interactions on the outcomes of chronic disease. *Med Care.* **27**(3): S110–27.

9   Steptoe A, Doherty S, Rink E *et al.* (1999) Behavioural counselling in general practice for the promotion of healthy behaviour among adults at increased risk of coronary heart disease: randomised trial. *BMJ.* **319**: 943–8.

10   Cegala D, Marinelli T and Post D (2000) The effects of patient communication skills training on compliance. *Arch Fam Med.* **9**: 57–64.

11   Kaplan SH, Gandez B, Greenfield S *et al.* (1995) Patient and visit characteristics related to physicians' participatory decision-making style. *Med Care.* **33**(12): 1176–87.

12   Chambers R and Wakley G (2000) *Making Clinical Governance Work for You.* Radcliffe Medical Press, Oxford.

13   Gillick v West Norfolk and Wisbech AHA (1985) **3** *All ER*: 402–37.

14   Department of Health (2000) *Contraceptive services for under 16-year olds: new guidance for health professionals.* Health Service Circular (in press). DoH, London.

15   Department of Health (1997) *Report on the Review of Patient-identifiable Information* (The Caldicott Committee report). Department of Health, London.

16   Wakley G, Chambers R and Field S (2000) *Continuing Professional Development in Primary Care: making it happen.* Radcliffe Medical Press, Oxford.

17   Mohanna K and Tunna K (1999) Withholding consent to participate in clinical trials: decisions of pregnant women. *Br J Obstet Gynaecol.* **106**: 892–7.

18   Lloyd AJ, Haynes PD, London NJ *et al.* (1999) Patients' ability to recall risk associated with treatment options. *Lancet.* **353**: 645.

19   James C (1999) Getting to grips with controlling demand. *Doctor.* **13 May**: 57–8.

20   Dakin G (2000) Appointments without a limit. *Medeconomics.* **April**: 48–50.

21   Chambers R (1998) *Clinical Effectiveness Made Easy.* Radcliffe Medical Press, Oxford.

22   Dolan P and Torgerson DJ (1998) The cost of treating osteoporotic fractures in the United Kingdom female population. *Osteoporos Int.* **8**: 611–17.

23   Torgerson DJ (1999) Cost-effectiveness of preventing osteoporotic fractures. *Osteoporos Rev.* **7**(3): 1–4.

24   Randall S, Webb A and Kishen M (1999) Presence of chaperone may interfere with doctor–patient relationship. *BMJ.* **319**: 1266 (letter).

25   Higson N (1996) *Risk Management: health and safety in primary care.* Butterworth-Heinemann, Oxford.

26   McCreadie C, Bennett G, Gilthorpe M *et al.* (2000) Elder abuse: do general practitioners know or care? *J R Soc Med.* **93**: 67–72.

27   Reason J (2000) Human error: models and management. *BMJ.* **320**: 768–70.

CHAPTER FIVE

Improving the explanation of risk: personal development plan

The future of continuing professional development in healthcare is likely to revolve around the construction of portfolios to demonstrate how we are keeping up to date. As a further illustration of how we can improve communication and explanation of risk, we give here an example of a personal development plan based on this topic.

This 'fictional' plan draws together some of themes discussed in Chapters 1 and 2. The template is offered as one that can be adapted for use with any topic.

Personal development plan: a worked example (the details should give you ideas – it is not intended to be comprehensive and particular pathways will be dependent on your personal needs)

What topic have you chosen: Risk

Who chose it?
I chose it for myself when I had a particularly difficult consultation with a patient who is a teacher who wanted to discuss whether she should start hormone replacement therapy or not.

Justify why topic is a priority:
A personal or professional priority?
I realise that I have a tendency to expect the patient to take my word for it when I explain why HRT is a 'Good Thing'. I'm making it a priority for myself to be able to explain risk

continued overleaf

better to patients and be able to make sense of the evidence in a way that balances risks against benefits. Also I need to be able to take the patient's perspective into account better so that the decision 'fits' with the way she looks at the world. I see it as a professional responsibility, like keeping up to date.

A practice priority?
I think there will be a spin-off from me looking into this that will help our practice nurse and health visitor as well. They occasionally have patients who query the need for immunisations for their children, for instance, and they usually refer the 'difficult' ones to me!

A national priority?
Risk is certainly on the national agenda at the moment what with the oral contraceptive pill scare for example. Risk management is one of the areas of clinical governance that we should all be addressing – not quite the same as communicating about relative risks, but some of the issues are the same like considering the patient's perspective for instance. The Department of Health is working on ways to improve risk communication with the public.

Who will be included in your personal development plan?

At the moment I think it is mostly an issue for me. I need to read a lot and get a better understanding of what the issues are. After that maybe I should start asking my partners what language they use to talk about risk and then involve patients to see how our advice is received. The nurses and health visitor should be involved since a lot of the discussion about immunisations and contraception takes place with them. Patients often ask the receptionists for advice when the mammography screening programme comes round, so maybe they should be included as well.

What baseline information will you collect and how?

A search of the literature will be important. I vaguely remember something in the *BMJ* about a risk scale a couple of years ago so I will dig that out and try to get some of the references at the end of that.

I could organise a very simple research project asking patients after consultations involving discussions of risk what their perceptions of the consultation had been. It could be a simple questionnaire. We could perhaps give it out at the baby clinic when the childhood immunisations are being given.

I would like to gather up examples of algorithms and graphs that help describe relative risks. I remember some in *Pulse*. The lab sent out some information on cardiovascular risk and lipids recently and there were some good colour graphs in a recent *BMJ* taken from Sheffield tables and New Zealand data which I could photocopy.

How will you identify your learning needs?

I will start keeping a diary – just jottings in surgery – about things that come up. If a patient asks, for example, for an estimate of his or her risk of a certain condition or the risks of a treatment option or screening test, and I find myself waffling or out of my depth, I will make a note. That way I can find out which areas I need to concentrate on.

continued opposite

If a patient comes back to see me or another partner after we have had a discussion, that will be useful feedback on how I explained things the first time.

I think the feedback from patients will be most useful. Maybe if the subject comes up with a patient I know well I could ask for their views at the end of the consultation when they have made a decision. A sort of informal 'how did I do?' approach.

I could also video-tape or audio-tape a few consultations and assess myself. The GP tutor will probably help go through them if I need a second opinion.

What are the learning needs for the practice and how do they match your needs?
It will be important to take into account the different consulting styles of the partners and nurses – after all, patients make a choice which one of us they come to see usually and that might have something to do with the differences between us. But at the same time it will be important that we have some standard way of explaining risk, especially if we are using scales or algorithms. The nurses will need to know how we are describing risk so that we can reinforce each other if a patient asks for a second opinion.

I don't know if the others will see it as a priority like I do – I will have to ask them.

Any patient or public input to your personal development plan?
The Patients' Association has done a lot on better communication in consultations and involving patients in discussions about care. I wonder if they have got anything on the language of risk? There is no sense reinventing the wheel if they have come up with good strategies or guidelines already.

Perhaps the surgery's patient participation group could have an item at one of their meetings when we can have an opportunity to discuss some of the more useful ways people at the surgery could help patients make informed decisions. If I decide to do a small survey to give me an idea about how things are at the moment it will be helpful to get their support and ideas.

I wonder if the Department of Public Health at the health authority has any papers on this?

Aims of your personal development plan arising from the preliminary data gathering exercise
By the end of the data collection period I should have an idea of:

1 those clinical areas of risk communication that I need to find out more about
2 patients' views on my strengths and weaknesses in communicating about risk
3 hints and suggestions about how others deal with this issue
4 the patients' perspective about how risk is best discussed
5 what graphs, aids and algorithms there are in the literature that might help me.

My personal development plan will have two main aims:

1 To develop a better understanding of the issues surrounding a discussion of risk and to help the rest of the practice team understand those issues.
2 To develop a resource for the practice library that contains aids for discussions with patients. These will be up-to-date and evidence-based so that everyone will have an answer if they are asked by a patient 'So how likely is that to happen to me?'

How might you integrate the 14 components of clinical governance?

Establishing a learning culture: Everyone is so busy that we don't really want to start having extra meetings to discuss this as people will just feel that it is another burden. I could use one of the regular practice meetings to talk about it and describe how I am keeping a notebook to jot down times when risk is discussed. I could suggest that the others try that as well and we could compare notes. This will get us all in the habit for when we start on our portfolios.

Managing resources and services: It makes sense that others in the team feel confident to discuss risks with patients, so that they don't have two appointments with different people when one will do. Also if some in the team turn out already to be better at it than others, we can share ideas.

Establishing a research and development culture: It will be a useful exercise to get to know the librarian at the postgraduate centre a bit better and use the resources there for the background reading. A survey of patients' views will be a good start to try and identify what the key issues are in risk communication. Perhaps if we find some algorithms that we think are useful we can actually test them out in a research project to see if they aid understanding in real life.

Reliable and accurate data: Part of the problem with talking about risk is that I don't really know some of the answers to patients' questions. It will be important to find out about the risks and benefits of things like HRT, keep up to date and make sure that discussions are evidence based.

Evidence-based practice and policy: Maybe risk communication could be something we build into the practice protocols as they come up for renewal. The ones on lipid-lowering drugs are due to be updated soon now that we have the new lab guidelines. We could have it as a section called something like 'explaining the risks and benefits to patients'. That way, with every area of clinical care that we consider, we will be looking at the literature for the evidence on risk/benefit. Involving patients in discussing the pros and cons of options will improve care.

Confidentiality: As always with individual patients, it is important to keep material about them confidential – even within the team. If we want to use individuals as a basis for discussion about risk it must all be anonymised. It is easy to assume information is safe in meetings but we should all bear this in mind.

Health gain: Better understanding of risk will lead to promotion of patients' autonomy, which should subsequently lead to health gains. Involving patients in discussions in an informed way about their health may lead to more responsibility for their health. A better understanding of the relative weight different risk factors have in the development of disease might also lead to more informed decision making. How many smokers request a cholesterol check for example? Being able to explain the whole picture of risk will avoid accusations that we are refusing blood tests because they cost too much and help patients understand the reasons decisions are made.

continued opposite

Coherent team: Some of us may already have good ways to describe risk to patients that we can share and the communication skills of some of us may be better. If we are all involved we can identify the strengths in the team. We will also provide a coherent message to patients if we have common ways to explain things.

Audit and evaluation: One way to evaluate how well we are getting on with an explanation of risk would be to repeat a survey similar to the assessment exercise with patients who have been shown the new risk communication aids to try and tease out whether their use has led to a better understanding of risk and more informed decision making.

Meaningful involvement of patients and the public: More informed individuals are more involved individuals, so by promoting discussion and shared decision making we are increasing individuals' involvement in their own care. Also the patient participation group will enjoy having something like this that they can get their teeth into, where we can demonstrate that their contribution is really needed and not being sought merely as a gesture.

Health promotion: Health promotion only works if patients really want to change. By improving the way we talk to patients about risk we should be able to reach a better understanding of the risks they face, from their lifestyle for example. I think patients get fed up if they perceive us as 'nagging' again, especially if we are offering advice that does not 'fit' with the way they look at the world or tally with their experience. By developing more of a joint discussion model we can encourage individual action. Undue pressure on patients to change doesn't work, but better explanation might.

Risk management: If patients play more of an active role in making decisions about their own health they will be less likely to blame us when it goes wrong! I think complaints arise out of failures of communication and that can include misunderstandings, for example about the limitations of treatments or the possibility of side effects. The main reason for having a good model for discussion of risk though is that it will enable us to effect change for our patients and hopefully improve outcomes. We need to be able to discuss things with those whose lifestyle is likely to be detrimental to their health in such a way that our words have an impact and result in change.

Accountability and performance: Performance will be much easier to maintain and monitor if we have developed protocols which everyone has had a share in and feels comfortable with using. It will be much less effective if I work alone, even if I am very enthusiastic!

Core requirements: Concentrating on risk communication in this way may identify team members whose communication skills are consistently remarked on by patients. Maybe we will see some training opportunities. I can already see that there may be a need for a team away-day where we can look at communication issues. Perhaps someone at the health authority could facilitate a session.

Action plan

Who is involved/setting: I think I will be taking the lead on this, especially with the background reading. I hope to include a representative from each group of health professionals, including the receptionists, in a working party though.

Timetabled action

First month: preliminary data gathering completed and staff involved:
- what light can the literature shed on the issues surrounding useful discussions of risk?
- what does the literature say on the subject of risk communication that will be useful for us?
- what communication aids are already available?
- ongoing log of areas that come up in consultation where I need to remedy my lack of knowledge.

By month three:
- complete the survey of health professionals' and patients' comments about risk
- video several consultations about risk to review my performance. Try to get objective feedback from patients and colleagues.

By month six: identify solutions and associated training needs:
- learn what barriers can exist to effective communication
- write or revise the practice protocols on the management of clinical conditions, taking into account the risk–benefit aspect for use in discussions with patients. Try to involve all the partners in the revisions and consult widely about the amendments
- consider team training in communication skills if appropriate, possibly externally mediated.

By end of the year: make changes:
- test out any new tools that we may have developed or discovered to see if they are actually effective in the consultation. Do they lead to a better understanding of risk and more informed decisions?
- consider sharing findings with other practices/members of the PCG
- could we publish any of our findings to reach a wider audience?

Expected outcomes: better and more fruitful communication with patients. More understanding of risk/benefit relationships for common therapeutic options (for both me and patients). Increased patient involvement in their care. Informed decision making by patients. Closer working relationships between team members and recognition of each others' areas of expertise.

How will you evaluate your personal development plan?
- Patient feedback.
- Critical review of performance.
- Repeat survey to complete the audit cycle.

How will you know when you have achieved your objectives?
My own understanding of risk will be improved so that I can help patients reach informed decisions. Discussion of risk will be easier aided by evidence-based protocols and better understanding of the facts. Patients will report greater involvement in decision making. Of course, I will have to ask them to know if I have achieved this!

How will you disseminate the learning from your plan to the rest of the practice team and patients? How will you sustain your newfound knowledge or skills?
The results will be disseminated by group involvement as we go along if I can continue to involve them and keep them interested. But it might be worth summing up the process by discussing the new protocols and decision aids in a regular practice meeting. I could also go back to the Patient Participation Group with the outcomes. I will make sure that protocol development/updating is on a rolling programme and that copies of everything are available in the library and for each consulting room.

How will you handle new learning requirements as they crop up?
I hope to keep my desktop log going in surgery so that I carry on jotting things down as I discover areas of poor knowledge, once I get into the habit. That way by a process of self-assessment and review of practice I can keep up to date. It will require a bit of self-discipline but once I get into the habit I expect the reading will actually be easier than at the moment because it will be more focused and I will be reading to find out specific answers.

Check out whether the topic you choose to learn is a priority and the way in which you plan to learn about it is appropriate

Your topic: Risk communication

How have you identified your learning need(s)?

a	PCG/T requirement	☐	e	Appraisal need	☐
b	Practice business plan	☐	f	New to post	☐
c	Legal mandatory requirement	☐	g	Individual decision	☒
d	Job requirement	☐	h	Patient feedback	☒
			i	Other	☐

Have you discussed or planned your learning needs with anyone else?
Yes ☒   No ☐   If so, who? Patients, team members, clinical tutor

What are the learning need(s) and/or objective(s) in terms of:
Knowledge: What new information do you hope to gain to help you do this?

Clearer understanding of the issues involved in a discussion of risk and how to hand this over most effectively to patients so that they can take more responsibility for decisions about their own health.

Skills: What should you be able to do differently as a result of undertaking this development?

Better communication about risk and more effective guiding of patients.

Behaviour/professional practice: How will this impact on the way you then do things?

It should keep us up to date and make us more coherent as a team.

Details and date of desired development activity:

• Within three months to finish the review of the literature and identify any risk communication tools that already exist.
• By the end of six months to have implemented the update of the clinical protocols incorporating risk/benefit assessment.
• By the end of the year to have piloted the use of the new decision aid in practice and evaluated its impact with a repeat patient survey.

Details of any previous training and/or experience you have in this area/dates:

None

Your current performance in this area against the requirements of your job:
Need significant development in this area ❑   Need some development in this area ☒
Satisfactory in this area   ❑   Do well in this area   ❑

Level of job relevance this area has to your role and responsibilities:
Has no relevance to job   ❑   Has some relevance   ❑
Relevant to job   ❑   Very relevant   ☒
Essential to job   ❑

Describe what aspect of your job and how the proposed education/training is relevant:
Helping patients make informed decisions about their health and trying to understand the choices they make in relation to other aspects of their life is an integral part of clinical practice. I can't believe it has taken me so long to realise that work needs to be done in this area!

Additional support in identifying a suitable development activity?
Yes ❑   No ☒

What do you need? N/A

Describe the differences or improvements for you, your practice, PCG/T and/or NHS Trust as a result of undertaking this activity?
I will have increased confidence in my ability to support, inform and guide patients. Patients will be more empowered, better informed and able to rely on more up-to-date facts about interventions. The team will be more integrated and better able to work together. Some of the antagonism some team members feel towards the patient participation group (that seems to come from a feeling that they are only interested in complaining about the service we provide) may be reduced.

Determine the priority of your proposed educational/training activity:
Urgent ❑   High ☒   Medium ❑   Low ❑

Describe how the proposed activity will meet your learning needs rather than any other type of course or training on the topic:
A course could help me learn more about risk, but only by reflecting on my practice and asking my patients will I understand what my strengths and weaknesses are and get some ideas about how to improve.

If you had a free choice would you want to learn this? Yes/No

If **no**, why not? (please circle all that apply):
    waste of time
    already done it
    not relevant to my work, career goals
    other

If **yes**, what reasons are most important to you (put in rank order):

improve my performance	1
increase my knowledge	2
get promotion	
just interested	4
be better than my colleagues	
do a more interesting job	5
be more confident	3
it will help me	

Record of your learning

Write in topic, date, time spent, type of learning

	Activity 1: literature review for information about risk	Activity 2: log book	Activity 3: survey of patients' views	Activity 4: update clinical protocols
In-house formal learning			Team discussion about questionnaire development	
External courses			May need some guidance on how to get best information from patients by interview or questionnaire	Keep an eye out for any update courses running locally on clinical issues
Informal and personal	Discuss with librarian how to use Medline Search for information explaining risk Look for risk communication tools	Get in the habit of jotting down areas that I find myself waffling about or unsure of the facts	Talk to individual patients in my surgery	Keep up to date with reading
Qualifications and/or experience gained	Understanding of issues surrounding the discussion of risk	Self-evaluation to find areas of clinical practice where I do not have enough knowledge of the facts	Patients' views about risk communication and examples of practice that help or get in the way of good understanding	Better baseline clinical knowledge to inform discussions with patients

CHAPTER SIX

Risk management: practice personal and professional development plan

Much of our continuing professional development will be based within a team setting. In general practice, the practice team will be expected to learn and develop together, building on the strengths of individual team members.

Just as Chapter 5 gave an example of a personal development plan, we have extended the topic of risk management to consider the construction of a practice personal and professional development plan. Again, the content of the plan draws together some of the themes from Chapters 3 and 4, but the template is offered as one that can be adapted for any subject area.

The relevance of this style of portfolio construction to the principles of clinical governance is highlighted by dividing up the plan according to the 14 subheadings of clinical governance referred to earlier.

Practice or workplace-based personal and professional development plan on risk management: a worked example (the details should give you ideas – it is not intended to be comprehensive and particular pathways will be dependent on your local situation and needs)

What topic: Risk management

Who chose it?
We chose it as a practice team; we all recognised that the topic was applicable to us in our roles as doctors, nurses, as a practice manager or as non-clinical staff.

Justify why topic is a priority

(i)   A practice priority? We may be putting patients at risk if their clinical management does not follow best practice; or if the practice organisation is inefficient and services or care are delayed or omitted. Patients and staff may be at risk if we do not adhere to legal requirements for health and safety issues.

(ii)   A district priority? Yes, effective risk management is core to addressing the clinical priorities in the district health improvement programme (HImP) – for instance coronary heart disease, diabetes and mental health care are priorities in the HImP. The PCG has made improving health and safety in its constituent practices a focus too, having found that many practices were breaching health and safety law when they visited individual practices across the PCG as part of their baseline assessment of clinical governance.

(iii) A national priority? Yes, risk management is central to the government's determination to guarantee minimum standards of care and services to everyone using the NHS. We should be able to reduce the chances of one of the practice team making an error to the detriment of patient care if we improve our risk management.

Who will be included in the practice-based plan?

We will include:
- practice nurses
- GPs
- practice manager
- receptionists
- practice secretaries
- cleaners
- local community pharmacists
- our two counsellors – voluntary, Relate
- community therapists
- health visitors
- district nurses
- social workers from our local patch

continued opposite

Who will collect the baseline information and how?

We will obtain information about the practice population and any needs assessments that have already been carried out from the public health department – our practice secretary will send for that – so that we can look to see if our services are broadly in line with our patients' needs and we are not neglecting any particular subgroup (e.g. non-English-speaking patients, people with particular chronic conditions).

We will run a computer search looking at how the medication we prescribe matches our practice protocols for three clinical conditions (hypertension, depression, hyperlipidaemia) backed up with audits to look at the length of treatment courses, frequency of review, identification of new cases, etc. One of our receptionists and the computer operator will do that.

The practice manager will review the extent to which we have been monitoring practice protocols and our records of risk assessment and risk reduction exercises in respect of health and safety in the practice.

Where are you now? (baseline)

This will include:

- a description of the practice population – numbers by age and gender; numbers of patients newly diagnosed in the past 12 months with the three clinical conditions we are focusing on: depression, hypertension and hyperlipidaemia. We should be able to retrieve this information in a computerised form; but we may find that various members of our practice team have been inconsistent about using Read codes and entering information about all clinical activities and consultations so we may need to use paper-based records to obtain this information as well
- comparison of prescribing in these three conditions; between us as prescribers in our practice; and between GPs in our practice and other practices. We hope that the local prescribing adviser will supply us with our prescribing patterns versus comparable anonymised PACT data from other practices
- referral patterns in the past 12 months for these three clinical conditions between our practice and other practices. The community psychiatric nurse, the PCG or health authority should be able to supply this comparative data
- we will look again at the results of the patient survey we did last year that enquired about patients' satisfaction and invited suggestions for improvements in relation to access, consultations with the doctor or nurse – the extent to which patients thought that we listened to them and explained matters
- we will undertake an audit looking at compliance with treatment and management. For example, the average length for which patients took medication or 'did not attend' figures for referrals to others (referrals between practice staff, and to counsellors, psychologists and psychiatrists for depression; numbers of patients who absconded from follow-up for hypertension and hyperlipidaemia)

continued overleaf

- we will consider undertaking a significant event audit where an adverse event actually happened or where there was a 'near miss'; and analyse what led up to those situations, and what lessons we can learn from them as a practice team
- we will find out what performance indicators are being used by the health authority or PCG that are being used to indicate the quality of care or services in local practices – and ask them for a copy of how we rate as individual GPs or the practice as a whole (e.g. comparative data on prescribing across the board, complaints, patients leaving our list but not moving house)
- we will map out numbers and types of staff with relevant expertise in our team: both employed staff members and those who are attached to the practice to whom we can refer patients – their particular skills and range of help offered. We will also list all the possible sources of help in the voluntary sector with their qualifications and expertise. This should help us to consider our options for delegation or exploring a different skill-mix or models of care in the practice when we try to improve the way we control risks.

What information will you obtain about individual learning wishes and needs?
Analysis of the significant event or critical incidents should enable the team to review what changes need to be made and which members of the practice team need further training to update their knowledge, skills or attitudes; or extend their capability for the planned changes in practice systems or procedures. For instance, we expect to look at a recent case where a young man committed suicide and in another incident, a patient with a history of hypertension had been lost to follow up and subsequently had a stroke. The staff involved may wish to update their clinical and interpersonal skills and, as depression and hypertension are our priority areas, we will support these areas of professional development in our practice learning plan.

We should be able to gauge which staff want to amend their roles and responsibilities and what is possible or realistic, by holding a practice team discussion that elicits people's concerns and their perceptions of the main issues for the practice in respect of clinical risk management.

All members of the practice will complete a check list that enquires about their specific needs; and give their views about the needs for improvement of other members of the team (e.g. Dr X does not refer appropriately to the CPN) or the practice organisation (e.g. communication between different members of staff about individual patients is poor). The practice manager might organise that.

The practice manager already discusses and agrees personal learning needs and goals with individual members of staff at their annual appraisals; the practice nurses have similar discussions in their clinical supervision and the GPs in our practice are setting up annual 'conversations' to discuss their personal development plans with the local GP tutor. We will feed these into the practice learning plan as appropriate.

continued opposite

What are the learning needs for the practice and how do they match the needs of the individual?

The practice nurses and the senior receptionist want to undertake accredited courses so that they have some transferable qualifications if they do move on in their careers or change practices. One of the practice nurse's aspirations matches the needs of the practice as she wishes to train as a nurse practitioner: and this will enable us to improve access for patients presenting with problems they perceive as being urgent. The second practice nurse wishes to update her knowledge of travel health; but we want her to attend an update course in mental healthcare instead so that she can absorb some of the patient workload of those who require counselling. The local Mental Health Trust is realigning the CPN's workload towards patients with severe and enduring mental illness so that we will have less available CPN time; and that practice nurse went on a travel health course last year.

The practice manager wants to attend courses on personal management skills – delegation and assertiveness; and organisational knowledge and skills – particularly to be updated on the new legal requirements for health and safety. The PCG is organising courses in all these topics and this will give our practice manager an opportunity to network with other local practices too – and exchange ideas on how they manage and control risks. The practice manager will then cascade his background knowledge and new learning to the rest of the practice team via a series of in-house meetings that explain and discuss revised practice protocols.

The GPs are all happy to prioritise the clinical conditions we have chosen to focus on in their personal development plans. As there are three GPs, each of us will take one of the three conditions for their own learning plan, that is relevant to the practice needs – so that each will subsequently take a lead in improving risk management for one of the priorities of depression, hypertension and hyperlipidaemia.

Any patient or public input to our plan?

We will ask patients with these three conditions about their care and seek their feedback on how we are doing; and ideas for improvements.

We will consult our patient panel to ask them for feedback about access and the appointment system, or suggestions for priority issues we might tackle – about the practice in general, or thinking of these three clinical conditions or health and safety aspects in particular.

We may invite one or two patients who suffer from one of the three clinical conditions we are focusing on to participate in our in-house training for staff to put the patient perspective and to keep us on track as a patient-centred practice.

How will you prioritise everyone's needs in a fair and open way?

We will gather all the available information and make it available to anyone working in the practice who is interested. We will finalise our practice-based learning plan at a designated practice team meeting where a representative of the nurses, GPs, practice staff and the practice manager attend. They will have talked to other staff members before the meeting so that they can relay and input their views.

continued overleaf

Objectives of the practice personal and professional development plan arising from the preliminary data gathering exercise

To identify and minimise clinical and organisational risks to patients and members of our practice in effective ways.

How you might integrate the 14 components of clinical governance into your practice-based professional development plan focusing on risk management

Establishing a learning culture: Designing the practice-based professional development plan through a democratic process; involving all relevant professionals, including attached staff (such as our community psychiatric nurse and community pharmacist) in practice-based teaching and learning.

Managing resources and services: Controlling how resources for training are allocated according to service-relevant needs; altering referral patterns according to agreed practice-based protocols for managing the three clinical conditions. Investing in equipment and furniture to comply with health and safety legislation (e.g. buying more sterilising equipment, wrist rests for typists, locks for cupboards).

Establishing a research and development culture: Encouraging all practice staff to critically appraise practice protocols as to whether they will achieve effective clinical management.

Reliable and accurate data: Agree ways of recording clinical conditions and information to which all staff adhere, e.g. use of Read codes; consistent entry on computer.

Evidence-based practice and policy: Individuals should be able to justify any deviations from the practice protocols for clinical matters in their consultations; adherence to health and safety law by all the practice team all the time.

Confidentiality: Increasing awareness of sharing and releasing information about a patient's medical details within the extended practice team on a 'need-to-know' basis.

Health gain: Increased staff awareness of the frequency with which depression presents with physical symptoms; increased staff expertise at detecting new cases of depression, hypertension and hyperlipidaemia.

Coherent team: Clearly agreed roles and responsibilities in management of these three clinical conditions and health and safety; and their underpinning systems and procedures. Everyone working within their areas of competence.

Audit and evaluation: Monitoring and review of success of the clinical and organisational risk management programmes taking account of the patient's circumstances and needs as well as clinical expertise.

Meaningful involvement of patients and the public: Developing meaningful methods of gaining patient input into the way the practice plans and delivers services, such as informal interviewing. Consult with voluntary organisations with a special interest in depression about how we may realistically improve our services for patients.

continued opposite

Health promotion: Screening of people for depression, hypertension and hyperlipidaemia – targeting high-risk groups such as those with diabetes or others who have had strokes.

Risk management: Anticipating those at risk of attempting suicide and taking preventive action whenever possible; reducing missed diagnoses of depression through improved expertise of all staff – clinicians and receptionists. Ensuring that risk reduction measures are bedded into our practice procedures following on from risk assessment of health and safety in our practice.

Accountability and performance: Collecting evidence of our problems and baseline measures so that others from outside the practice may judge our improved performance as individuals and as a practice team.

Core requirements: Including time and support for members of the practice team to prevent them from becoming depressed or burnt out in response to the volume of work, frequent changes and competing service demands. We will work towards developing practice systems and procedures that are cost and time effective.

Action plan

Who is involved/setting: All staff as set out above.

Timetabled action: Start date

By three months: preliminary data gathering completed:
- each GP leading on the clinical topic of depression, hypertension and hyperlipidaemia and the practice manager leading on health and safety will review the practice protocols (including clinical management and the underpinning systems and procedures). We will check that they are up to date and conform to recently published best practice. Everyone's roles and responsibilities should be clearly laid out. We will consider the extent to which practice protocols fit with others' management plans (e.g. a PCG-sponsored template for health and safety across all constituent practices, care pathways for the local hospital trust)
- list numbers of staff; map expertise completed; describe other providers of healthcare available in the locality
- GP leads look at referral and prescribing patterns in respect of the three conditions
- gather information about the characteristics of practice population, our performance, relevant local and national priorities – organised by one of the practice nurses
- staff complete checklists giving views and suggestions about their training needs, ways to improve services – organised by practice manager
- obtain any relevant performance indicators held by the PCG or the health authority – one of the GPs who is on the PCG board to do this.

By six months: review current performance:
- monitor the extent of our knowledge and adherence to practice protocols for managing the three priority clinical conditions and health and safety – GPs and practice manager lead and delegate audits and data collection to non-clinical staff

continued overleaf

- monitor access to appointments, telephone advice – audit of actual performance via pre-agreed criteria – focusing too on any particular subgroups of patients who might have particular difficulties, such as elderly people or the housebound. Organised by practice manager and delegated to others in practice team
- discuss results of recent or current audits (including significant event audit as described earlier) in practice team meeting
- compare our performance in relation to at least four of the 14 components of clinical governance previously described.

By nine months: identified solutions and associated training needs:
- set up new systems for appropriate triage of priority patients by the receptionists and practice nurses – agreed in practice team meetings
- GP leads or practice manager to have written or revised practice protocols as appropriate, having searched for other evidence-based protocols; with input from others in secondary care, the practice team, attached staff and patients
- identified gaps in care or hazards, and proposed changes to delivery of care or services so that GPs and nurses adhere to revised practice protocols that minimise the probability of risks occurring, or reduce the impact on patients or the practice if they do
- GPs, nurses and practice manager to have agreed revised roles and responsibilities of practice team for improving delivery of care and services that minimise risks occurring in clinical management of the three priority clinical conditions or other clinical matters, or health and safety
- certain staff attend external courses or in-house training as appropriate to practice-based learning plan; for instance, receptionists have in-house training on triage
- one GP to have liaised with GP co-operative to review how GP deputies and nurses triage calls from or about those at high risk of these priority clinical conditions or others. If widespread learning need contact GP tutor to request series of district-based seminars.

By 12 months: make changes:
- practice manager feeds back information to PCG and trust to justify request for more resources
- improve access, find ways to prioritise patients at high risk; improve security of records and confidentiality of patients' medical details
- practice manager to buy new equipment to minimise health and safety risks, e.g. to enhance personal safety of individuals of practice team.

Expected outcomes: more effective risk management of depression, hypertension and hyperlipidaemia; better patient compliance with medication and attendance at referrals; more flexible access arrangements. No or infrequent breaches of health and safety legislation. More consistent use of Read codes by all practice team members.

How does your learning plan tie in with your other strategic plans?
Managing risk should be a priority for the practice business and development plan too as the great deal of effort to be expended on improving the care and services is likely to absorb significant time and resources.

The PCG has nominated health and safety in general practices as a priority for the current year's operation – in terms of training and reimbursement of costs.

Our practice aims to work more closely with the local hospital trust to provide more seamless care for patients crossing the primary–secondary care interface: this plan should result in a more coordinated approach by using practice protocols that complement those on the hospital side; so reducing risks arising from confusion and inconsistencies between the primary and secondary care sectors.

What additional resources will you require to execute your plan and from where do you hope to obtain them?
We will require resources for training, changing prescribing and referral patterns (this might be an extra cost justified by health gains or cost savings). We will realign our current resources or seek additional support from the PCG; as we are focusing on priorities in the district's and the PCG's strategic plans, we may be able to tap into any additional resources that are available.

How much protected time will you allocate to staff to undertake the learning described in your plan?
This will depend on their circumstances, aspirations and needs that arise when formulating and undertaking the action plan.

How will you evaluate your learning plan? (who will be responsible for what?)
By analysing our strengths, weaknesses, opportunities and threats (SWOT) as a practice in providing care for those with depression, hypertension and hyperlipidaemia after we have completed our action plan, so we can see what we have achieved and what is left to do.

We will use audit to compare the baseline assessment and progress at the completion of the initiative against our set standards – for health and safety as well as the three priority clinical conditions.

How will you know when you have achieved your objectives?
Using the audit and survey methods described above and measuring deviation from the agreed practice protocols.

How will you handle new learning requirements as they crop up?
The practice manager who leads the initiative will collate suggestions, complaints and observations as they are made by staff or patients in response to the new systems. The practice manager, clinical supervisor and GP tutor will revisit the topic of risk management in annual appraisals to check on progress and any perceived new learning requirements.

Record of practice team learning about risk management

	Activity 1: depression	Activity 2: hypertension	Activity 3: hyperlipidaemia	Activity 4: health and safety
In-house formal learning	Community psychiatric nurse holds one-hour lunchtime session with all practice team – highlighting types of high-risk patients, discussing triage and recommended action	Community pharmacist and GP lead in practice for hypertension facilitate one-hour lunchtime session with GPs and practice nurses reviewing prescribing patterns and discussing best practice	Practice nurse and GP lead in practice for hyperlipidaemia feed back results of audits of high-risk patients and discuss standards set in National Service Framework for coronary heart disease	PCG-organised facilitator visits practice to run training session for all the practice team. Staff from two local single-handed practices join in; update on current legal requirements and practical advice
External courses	GP lead and one of the practice nurses attends a day-long update course at local Mental Health Trust. Input from voluntary sector	GP lead and one of the practice nurses attends a half-day update course organised at local postgraduate centre	GP lead and one of the practice nurses attends a half-day update course organised at local postgraduate centre	
Informal and personal	GP lead reads several published papers from medical journals on best practice and reflects on how own practice matches up	Discussions with others at update course about how they identify new hypertensives and manage high-risk patients	Several chats at coffee breaks in the practice between GPs, practice nurses and district nurses about which patients the practice should be targeting lipid management at	Practice manager does exchange visit with another practice manager where each informally inspects the other to check whether the practice is breaching health and safety law in any way
Qualifications and/or experience gained	Evidence of portfolio ready for revalidation	Evidence for portfolio ready for revalidation	Evidence for portfolio ready for revalidation	Evidence for any future external inspection of health and safety; evidence for portfolio ready for revalidation of doctors

Appendix: Sources of further information

General information

For doctors seeking authoritative information, or places to which they can direct their patients, links to reviewed websites can be found at the **Doctors Net UK** website. This medical Internet company reviews all sites quoted on their website and can be reached at www.doctors.net.uk or fax: 01235 862791.

National Freephone Health Information Service (tel: 0800 665544). Patients can often find answers to simple questions at this health authority information service. Each authority is obliged to provide access to such a service and although the details will vary from one area to another there are national guidelines about access and the type of information available.

NHS Direct (tel: 0845 4647). Staffed by nurses, this 24-hour telephone information service can also provide answers or advice about contacting medical services. As a further part of NHS Direct, NHS Direct On-Line is being developed for patients and the public at the National Electronic Library for Health (www.nelh.nhs.uk/). Designed to give easy access to information the service aims to help patients address three questions:

- How can I stay healthy and reduce my risk of disease?
- Should I see my doctor?
- Am I getting the right type of care and treatment for my health problem?

Help for Health Trust (tel: 01962 849100; www.hfht.demon.co.uk/). This service is based in Winchester and provides information as part of the Health Information Service and NHS Direct for Hampshire. This trust runs a consumer health information library and database, including 'Helpbox', a source of details about national self-help groups and references to self-help literature on a wide range of health issues.

HebsWeb (www.hebs.scot.nhs.uk/) is the website for the Health Education Board of Scotland; a popular site providing access to a wide range of consumer health information and resources through a virtual health centre.

HPIC Health Promotion Information Centre (www.hea.org.uk.hpic/) is the national centre for health promotion information and advice in England and part of the Health Development Agency. It includes access to databases covering a variety of health issues and topics in a range of formats.

Medline Plus (www.nlm.nih.gov/medlineplus/) is supported by the US National Library of Medicine and provides access to a wide range of databases, including the abstracts of articles indexed on Medline.

National Institutes of Health (www.nih.gov/health/consumer/) provides access to databases of consumer health information published by the US National Institutes of Health. The NIH search engine is also available.

Patient UK (www.patient.co.uk/) is designed to direct non-medical people in the UK to information about health-related issues and is maintained by two general practitioners responsible for the patient information leaflet service (PILS).

www.betterhealth.com/virtualcheckup/noplugin/heart/index.html invites consumers to input data relating to their cardiovascular health, such as blood pressure and cholesterol concentration. The site then gives an assessment coupled with a diagram of the coronary arteries. For curious patients this has novelty value but clearly must be accompanied by medical advice.

One British site answers medical questions over the web. www.netdoctor.co.uk carries a disclaimer stating that the site is designed to support not replace the doctor–patient relationship, but offers counselling, advice and information in response to individual patient inquiries.

Directories of self-help groups can help newly diagnosed patients find support. Two good UK sites that can help are www.cafamily.org.uk/home.html and http://www.patient.co.uk A similar American based resource is at www.healthy.net/home/index.html

www.medicdirect.co.uk was founded by an ENT surgeon in Birmingham and aims to present simple information to supplement that given by their GP. In particular, the aim is to raise awareness on issues such as breast and testicular examination, which some people may feel reluctant to discuss with their own GP.

Quality issues

The Centre for Health Information Quality (tel: 01962 863511; enquiries@ centreforhiq.demon.co.uk; www.centreforhiq.demon.co.uk/) is funded by the NHS Executive as a central resource to facilitate the production and dissemination of high-quality patient information for health service users. This service does not currently provide access to information on specific conditions or treatments, but provides advice on quality guidelines and initiatives and works directly with NHS and patient representatives to raise awareness of key issues in the development of consumer health information.

DISCERN (www.discern.org.uk) is an instrument developed to assess the quality of health information on treatment choices. A number of hints are given after each question to guide the user. Areas covered are: bias in the material, a clear statement of aims, references and additional sources of support and information, uncertainty, risks and benefits (including those of opting for no treatment), and treatment options. DISCERN also alerts the user to concepts such as shared decision making and quality of life. It has already been widely validated for written leaflets and for use by designers of new information as well as people assessing existing material.

Gateway sites

For those patients or doctors not knowing quite where to start in the quest for information a gateway to other directories can be found at http://www.lib.uiowa.edu/hardin/md/index.html This site is catalogued by specialty and can guide users to other sources of information.

Other 'gateway sites' can also help guide searches often by supplying links to other websites.

Healthfinder (www.healthfinder.gov/) is a US government site that provides access to health information from a range of sources, including government agencies, voluntary groups and professional organisations. It has links to Medline Plus and other online databases.

Health On the Net (HON) Foundation (www.hon.ch/) provides a database of evaluated health materials and also promotes the use of the HON code as a self-governance initiative to help unify the quality of medical and health information available. Users of website health information displaying the HON logo can be assured that the material has been developed in accordance with these guidelines.

Organising Medical Networked Information (OMNI) (www.omni.ac.uk) is based at the University of Nottingham and provides access to good-quality biomedical and health information from the Internet worldwide. It has been developed primarily for medical professionals, but consumers may find it useful.

Sites for specific conditions

Cancer

Cancer Help UK is at http://medweb.bham.ac.uk/Cancerhelp/indexg.html Based at the University of Birmingham in the Cancer Research Campaign's Institute of Cancer Research, this is a very user-friendly and comprehensive site for this massive topic.

CancerBacup, a site that caters for both doctors and patients, is at www.cancerbacup. org.uk This UK-based resource on cancer information and support is aimed primarily at people with cancer and their families or carers but has separate sections for health professionals and patients.

The welcome page for the **Philippine Breast Cancer Network** (http://pbcn.findhere. com) introduces a patient pressure group. The site contains personal histories of women with breast cancer that some patients may find supportive.

Impotence

A branch of the US-based **National Institutes of Health** has produced a publication on impotence for doctors and patients (www.niddk.nih.gov/health/urolog/pubs/impotence/ impotence.htm). Since the page is copyright-free, material can be downloaded and photocopied in the surgery.

The Risk Ready Reckoner©

Risk factor (reference)	Risk estimate	Verbal scale	Comparator (in UK)
All natural causes risk of death aged 40 [4]	1 in 850	Moderate	Like one person in a village
Risk of dying in any one year from smoking 10 cigarettes per day [4]	1 in 200	Moderate	
Lifetime risk of cancer (any type) [9]	1 in 3	Very high	
Breast cancer in women [7]			
– lifetime risk	8 in 100	High	Like a three-ball win on the lottery
– baseline expected risk aged 50–75	45 in 1000	Moderate	
– on HRT for 5 years	47 in 1000	Moderate	
– on HRT for 10 years	51 in 1000	Moderate	
– on HRT for 15 years	57 in 1000	Moderate	
Osteoporosis			
– lifetime risk of a 50-year-old woman [5]	4 in 10	Very high	
– lifetime risk for men	13 in 100	High	
– risk of hip fracture if on HRT	13 in 100	High	
Cardiovascular risk			
– event in next five years for a non-smoker aged 50 [6]	47 in 100	High	
– on HRT for 5 years	36 in 100	High	
Ovarian cancer [3]			
– baseline risk aged 45	1 in 10 000	Low	Like the risk of death per year in pregnancy
– with an affected sister	5 in 100	High	
– with an affected mother	7.5 in 100	High	

continued opposite

Risk factor (reference)	Risk estimate	Verbal scale	Comparator (in UK)
Oral contraceptive pill (OCP)			
– death (non-smoker, under 35) [2]	1 in 77 000	Very low	Like the risk of being a murder victim
– thrombosis [1]	15 in 100 000	Low	Like the risk of dying in a car accident
– baseline risk of thrombosis (not on pill) [1]	5 in 100 000	Very low	Like the risk of a man dying in a soccer accident
– thrombosis on third generation OCP [2]	30 in 100 000	Low	Like death from any kind of violence or poisoning
– breast cancer aged 45 with 5 years on OCP [10]	11.1 in 1000	Moderate	
– baseline risk aged 45 with no OCP use [10]	10 in 1000	Moderate	
Pregnancy in the UK [8]			
– death from all causes	1 in 10 000	Low	Like one in a small town
– deep venous thrombosis [1]	60 in 100 000	Low	
– miscarriage	1 in 4	Very high	
– congenital abnormality	2 in 100 births	High	
Amniocentesis [8]			
– discovery of an abnormality	1 in 600 tests	Moderate	The risk of death per year for hang gliders
– miscarriage	1 in 100	Moderate	Like the risk of dying from smoking 15 cigarettes per day
Risks of other medical intervention			
– contracting HIV infection from donated blood	1 in 2 500 000	Negligible	Like a six-ball win (jackpot) on the lottery

continued overleaf

Risk factor (reference)	Risk estimate	Verbal scale	Comparator (in UK)
Risks of other medical intervention (cont)			
– contracting hepatitis C from donated blood	1 in 300 000	Minimal	Like the risk of dying in a railway accident
– additional lifetime risk of fatal cancer from abdominal CT [9]	1 in 2000	Low	Like an extra 4.5 years of background radiation
– additional lifetime fatal cancer risk resulting from a chest X-ray examination [9]	1 in 1 000 000	Negligible	Like an extra three days of natural background radiation

1 *Drugs and Therapeutics Bulletin* (2000) Oral contraceptives and cardiovascular risk. **38**(1): 1–5.
2 Calman K (1996) Cancer: science and society and the communication of risk. *BMJ*. **313**: 799–802.
3 Stratton JF et al. (1998) A systematic review and meta-analysis of family history and risk of ovarian cancer. *Br J Obstet Gynaecol*. **105**: 493–9.
4 Henderson M (1990) *The BMA Guide to Living with Risk*. Penguin, Harmondsworth.
5 Grady D et al. (1992) Hormone therapy to prevent disease and prolong life in postmenopausal women. *Ann Int Med*. **117**: 1016–37.
6 Anderson KV et al. (1991) Cardiovascular disease risk profiles. *Am Heart J*. **121**: 203–8.
7 Collaborative Group on Hormonal Factors in Breast Cancer (1997) Breast cancer and hormone replacement therapy: collaborative reanalysis of data from 51 epidemiological studies of 52,705 women with breast cancer and 108,411 women without breast cancer. *Lancet*. **350**(9084): 1047–59.
8 Cusick W and Vintzileos AM (1999) Fetal Down's syndrome screening: a cost effectiveness analysis of alternative screening programs. *J Matern Fetal Med*. **8**(6): 243–8.
9 The Royal College of Radiologists (1998) *Making the Best Use of Department of Radiology Guidelines for Doctors* (4e). The Royal College of Radiologists, London.
10 Guillebaud J (1997) *Contraception Today* (3e). Martin Dunitz, London.

Index